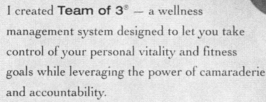
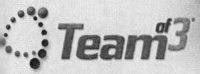

To Coach Ben Parks,

who mentored me for eighteen years
with values and integrity that have become the
foundation of my life's work in the fitness industry.

Because of your influence in my life,
thousands of people also call me Coach.
To you, I am forever grateful.

Published in Nashville, Tennessee, by Thomas Nelson, Inc.

Nelson Books titles may be purchased in bulk for educational, business, fund-raising, or sales promotional use. For information, please e-mail SpecialMarkets@ThomasNelson.com.

Scripture references noted NKJV are from THE NEW KING JAMES VERSION. Copyright © 1979, 1980, 1982, Thomas Nelson, Inc., Publishers.

Scripture references noted NIV are from the HOLY BIBLE: NEW INTERNATIONAL VERSION®. Copyright © 1973, 1978, 1984 by International Bible Society. Used by permission of Zondervan Publishing House. All rights reserved.

Library of Congress Cataloging-in-Publication Data

Nava, Don.
    Fit after 40 : 3 keys to looking good and feeling great / Don Nava.
      p. cm.
    ISBN: 978-0-7852-9786-4
    1. Middle-aged persons--Health and hygiene. 2. Middle-aged persons--Psychology. 3. Physical fitness for middle-aged persons. 4. Exercise for middle-aged persons. I. Title: Fit after forty. II. Title.
    RA777.5.N38 2006
    613'.0434--dc22
                              2005035681

Printed in the United States of America
06 07 08 09 QW 1 2 3 4 5 6

FIT
AFTER
40

3 keys to looking good and feeling great

Coach Don Nava

THOMAS NELSON PUBLISHERS
Nashville

A Division of Thomas Nelson, Inc.

For other life-enriching books, visit us at:
www.thomasnelson.com

CONTENTS

CHAPTER 1

The Magical Milestone Birthday

Midlife is real. Nobody seems to know the exact age range it should cover, but everybody I know has a sense about when they are—or aren't—in the middle of what they perceive to be a normal life span. People seem intuitively to know when they are in their early years, when they are in their later years, and when they are someplace in between.

Midlife crises are also real. Again, nobody seems to know exactly *when* a midlife crisis normally hits. But there's a moment when the light comes on and you say, *Yikes, I'm not getting any younger!*

The trigger point might be a little pain or stiffness that wasn't there before.

The trigger point might be a failure to do something that was once so easy.

The trigger point might be an "Oh, Dad" or "Oh, Mom" roll of the eyes after you say something that seems totally rational and normal from your perspective.

The trigger point might be the day a clerk asks if you qualify for a senior-citizen discount (and you thought that day was ten years away); or the time you hear yourself say, "Kids these days—" with an exasperated sigh; or the time you begin to remember with fondness the "good ol' days" when you were thirty-something.

The trigger point might be the wrinkles you see in the mirror, the gray hair that suddenly seems to be multiplying, or the nagging thought that you probably *should* go see a doctor more frequently, but have less and less desire to do so out of fear that something bad might be discovered.

The trigger point can be any one of a number of physical or emotional cues that are unique to each person.

The "crisis" is, in part, a facing of one's own mortality. It occurs, in part, because the person recognizes that there are still things he or she *wants* to do, accomplish, or experience. Stop and think about it—if you've done or are in the process of doing everything you dream of doing, and are as happy as you want to be, there's no real sense of crisis! The crisis can be a slight moment of panic or a major period of panic—either of which is rooted in an unhappy, unfulfilled feeling.

The crisis often prompts a person to make an attempt to regain some sense of control over his destiny, or some sense of control over his "happiness level." Not every person openly acknowledges or even recognizes that a crisis is occurring—some people just have a nagging, persistent feeling deep within that if the time is ever going to be right to make a move or make a change, that time is now.

Reactions to midlife crises vary, of course. I'm in the total-fitness business, and I've seen some people go off the deep end.

Some people go a step or two beyond crazy and immediately *try* to dress and act twenty years younger. I put emphasis on *try* because they rarely succeed. The clothes of the younger generation look a little silly on them, their hair dye is never quite color-perfect, the "teen" phrases coming out of their mouths sound very odd, and their behavior at the "in places" is usually regarded by the younger set as both obvious and bizarre.

I have nothing against motorcycles or skydiving, but if the purpose is to prove that a person is still young, the end result is more likely to be raised eyebrows than sincere applause.

At the other end of the midlife crisis spectrum are those who plop themselves down to await the arrival of the grim reaper. In doing so, they begin to act and think much older than their years. They curl up in an overstuffed recliner before inane television programs and gorge themselves on fast-food specials. They stop taking risks of any kind and cease to foster their own curiosity or sense of adventure. They conclude that they've "been there, done that" about virtually everything fun or meaningful in life.

And in truth, the more they harden themselves into "thinking" like an old person, the sooner they bring about their own demise—perhaps not necessarily their own death, but with certainty, their own decline in productivity, creativity, and sense of purpose.

There are a host of reactions to midlife that fall someplace between trying too hard to be young and unwittingly falling into acting too old. Most of the reactions are just plain stupid because they are totally unnecessary and counterproductive to a joyful life. A few reactions are legitimate and productive.

This book focuses on the *positive* and beneficial reactions to midlife that can turn a crisis moment into a creative, compelling moment of change and growth.

YOUR MAGICAL MILESTONE BIRTHDAY

Whichever birthday it is for you, you either have had or will have what I call a "magical milestone birthday." It is the birthday when you say, "I can't believe I'm this age."

For some that age is thirty. For some it is fifty. For some it is sixty. For lots of people the magical milestone birthday is forty, and that's why this book addresses living a Totally Fit Life after the age of forty. There's something about the age of forty that seems to mark a passing from youth. A friend of mine said not too long ago, "I knew I was in midlife when I noticed that I was helping to plan an all-day church picnic and I was calling people twenty years younger than me 'the young people' and people twenty years older than me 'the older set.'" Her mind-set covered forty years.

In the Bible, a generation is considered to be forty years in length. Perhaps people intuitively feel that when they hit forty, they move into the "older generation"—the one previously occupied by their parents.

As we were discussing this concept of a forty-year mark, another friend said: "I never really felt any different when I hit forty, but I did notice that other people started to pay more attention to my opinions when I spoke up at meetings. I was taken more seriously after I turned forty. My father told me that when he turned eighty, he suddenly was treated with greater respect. He could get away with a lot of things that people wouldn't tolerate when he was sixty or seventy."

If the year isn't exactly forty for you, then name your year. There's *one* birthday that you'll see as a threshold or a "line in the sand" that you are about to cross.

The question is, How do you cross that line? Do you go crazy, or go comatose?

I like the concept "captivate."

CHOOSE TO CAPTIVATE

The original definition of the word *captivate* means to take something captive, and then to hold on to that something by irresistibly positive and pleasing means.

Rather than be taken captive by the passing of years, choose to recapture your life and future! Choose to take captive the moments of each day and the days of each year. Choose to hold on to your own sense of identity by making positive decisions and taking positive action. Choose to fulfill your purpose for living in a way that gives you maximum satisfaction and joy.

If you need to reinvent yourself to find fulfillment, do so in a way that is healthful and helpful not only to you but also to others around you.

If you need to refocus your goals toward a new and higher purpose, do so with wise counsel.

If you need to resculpt your out-of-shape body for greater health, do so with good eating, good exercising, and good coaching.

If you need to reinvigorate relationships that have fallen into a rut, do so with enthusiasm and love.

If you need to reestablish or renew your faith—do so.

If you need to refocus or readjust your schedule, expenditures of time and money, or material possessions to achieve something that is in line with your highest values and beliefs, do so.

Captivate! Grab hold of your life. In some cases, you'll be putting on the brakes; in others, you'll be pressing down on the accelerator. In some cases, you'll be getting in gear; in other cases moving to a higher gear. In some cases you'll be steering your life in a new direction, and in some cases slowing down to enjoy the scenery.

The captivate process is slightly different for each person, but the end goal is the same—a life that is more balanced, enjoyable, and fulfilling.

LONGER LIFE OR HIGHER QUALITY?

I'm not at all certain that we can make changes that will impact the number of years we live. What I am certain about is this: we *can* impact the *quality* of life we enjoy, both now and in the future.

Every person I have ever met *can* make decisions that have a high probability of producing more energy, vitality, and health in the future.

A person *can* make decisions that hold the potential for increased fulfillment and purpose.

A person *can* make choices that result in greater integrity, deeper character, and an even more positive reputation and legacy.

A person *can* make decisions that promote deeper relationships and more influence for good in any given family, group, community, society, or the world as a whole.

You may not be able to add years to your life, but you most certainly *can* add life to your years.

There is a tremendous opportunity that awaits you as you cross a magical milestone birthday. Choose to take captive every thought, every word, and every deed that might *add* life to your years. A great deal of healthy, purposeful, important living can occur *after* that birthday comes and goes.

CHAPTER 2

In Pursuit of the Totally Fit Life

I frequently have the opportunity to speak to Christian church groups and men's retreats. A question I enjoy asking is, "Are you living an abundant life?" A few hands might go up, but very tentatively. A few people might have an inkling about what I'm asking, but most don't. The great majority of people have either puzzled or ashamed looks on their faces.

I then read what Jesus said: "The thief does not come except to steal, and to kill, and to destroy. I have come that they may have life, and that they may have it more abundantly" (John 10:10 NKJV).

I usually say to the group: "I don't think Jesus would have told us He came to give us something that we can't receive, do, or enjoy. *Abundance* refers to an overflowing amount of everything that is beneficial to life— health, vitality, energy, strength, purpose, ministry effectiveness, career success, fulfillment, finances, friendships, loving family relationships, intellectual growth, and emotional well-being.

"Not only does abundance refer to an overflowing *quantity* of these good things—and many other good things—but also to having these things in balance. The Jewish understanding of wholeness was that all aspects of life are both present and balanced. So let me ask you again: Are you truly living an abundant life?"

Most of the time, no hand is raised. The follow-up question is then, "But how many of you *want* to live an abundant life—all things that are beneficial and good being present and balanced in your life?"

Every hand goes up! Everybody *wants* to be whole. Everybody *wants* to have their priorities in the right order. Everybody *wants* to enjoy a life that is filled to overflowing with health, joy, purpose, fulfillment, and blessings.

But how?

For me, the first step is a practical one in defining what it means to live an abundant life, or a "whole" life. I call the life we all desire the "Totally Fit Life."

"ARE YOU TALKING ABOUT EXERCISE?"

I had spent more than an hour describing the Totally Fit Life to a group, with a few questions and answers afterward. Lucille hadn't heard any of it, or so it seemed. She came to me after the presentation and asked: "Are you talking about exercise?"

I said, "You hate to exercise, don't you?"

She looked at me a little skeptically, perhaps trying to figure out if I was a mind reader. "How did you know?"

I laughed. "Because you wouldn't have zeroed in on that one aspect of a Totally Fit Life if you didn't know, at least subconsciously, that you *aren't* doing the one thing you *should* be doing. The main reason people don't usually *do* what they know they *should* do is because they hate doing it."

She looked puzzled. "Lucille," I continued, "everybody does what they choose to do. Most of our choices are based on what we *like* to do. That's human nature. We know we shouldn't eat two rich chocolate desserts in one day but hey, we like chocolate and we tell ourselves that desserts like that don't come along very often, so we eat them.

"If someone comes along and says, 'You shouldn't eat chocolate,' you may know he's right, but you don't want to hear that message, or even worse, you decide you don't like him for speaking the truth. The person can tell you not to do a dozen other things, but the only thing you hear is 'you shouldn't eat chocolate'—because that's your downfall."

She nodded in agreement.

"Here's the real clincher," I continued. "Ninety-nine out of a hundred people focus on the one thing that keeps them from being whole more than they focus on the many other things they are doing that contribute to their wholeness."

"We see the fly in the soup," she said.

I laughed. "That's not exactly the example I would have chosen," I said, "but you're right. We intuitively, instinctively know the problem area in our life. We focus on the thing we don't do because we hate to do it. We throw out the entire concept of total fitness because we just don't think we can—or don't *want*—to do the one thing we dislike. The good news is that you've recognized you don't like to exercise."

"You're right," she said. "That's the one part of my life I know I should do, but I hate to do it, so I don't do it. It's the reason I'm in the shape I'm in."

I knew it wasn't the only reason, but that was going to be another conversation.

I asked, "You like people, don't you?"

"Sure," she said.

"You have good friendships and good relationships with people at work, right?"

"I do," she said.

"You feel good about your purpose in life and the type of work you do?"

"I do," she said.

"You have a solid spiritual life and are involved in at least one activity that you know is helping someone in need?"

"Yes," she said. "I'm active in my church, and I help with the program that prepares lunch for the homeless people in our area."

"Are you learning and growing mentally?" I asked.

"Actually, I just began taking a course at the local junior college," she said. "I love it."

"So it's just the exercising that keeps your from a Totally Fit Life?" I asked.

"I guess so."

"Well, I have great news! That's the easiest part to get back into balance. And furthermore, you *can* learn to like exercising, so much so that you won't want to go more than a day or two without it."

"You're kidding," Lucille said candidly. I liked Lucille. She didn't waste words.

"Yes," I said, "I guarantee it. Give me a ten-week commitment to exercising, and I'll show you a way to enjoy it and get the most out of it."

"You're on," she said, and we set up a phone appointment time.

What was encouraging in that brief encounter with Lucille was that, even though she was in her fifties, she had come to a meeting titled "Exploring the Totally Fit Life." She wanted something she knew she didn't have.

I was also encouraged that she already knew and had owned up to what was keeping her from being totally fit. Many people don't know, or don't want to own up to the "missing ingredient" that is keeping them from total fitness. Do you?

- What one thing do you believe keeps you from experiencing a Totally Fit Life?
- Why is this a problem area for you?

- What don't you like to do or don't want to do?
- Are you willing to admit that this is the one area of your life in which you should take action?

During my second conversation with Lucille, she admitted to me that she was fifty-two years old, hadn't exercised since she was twenty-three, and hated to perspire. She had never belonged to a gym and didn't really want to go to one. She thought she might enjoy walking, however, and she agreed that it would be more fun to walk with someone. She agreed that she'd work with me for ten weeks on a specified set of goals, and that we'd reevaluate things after that.

A large number of people from the presentation at Lucille's church submitted cards on which they indicated their exercise preferences, availability for exercise, and their willingness to have an exercise partner. I hooked up Lucille with Ramona, another woman in her church, who was fifty-one and liked to exercise. Ramona enjoyed walking and thought it might be good to walk with someone regularly.

Ramona's marriage had just ended in a messy divorce, and she was ashamed to be divorced. As a Christian she believed divorce was wrong, and she thought other people in the church might be looking down on her for being divorced, even though nothing about the breakup of her marriage had been her idea. She had low self-esteem, was incapable of trusting very many people, and felt discouraged and even a little depressed on most days. Lucille didn't have any of those problems but could empathize.

The two of them made an agreement—they were going to become totally fit. For Lucille, that meant exercising and learning to like it. For Ramona, the Totally Fit Life meant regaining her balance emotionally and directionally.

I gave both of these women information that covered the basics of the Totally Fit Life. A few of those basics follow.

A Balanced Whole

The Totally Fit Life encompasses six areas of life intended to be viewed as a balanced whole:

1. *Physical*—including general health habits and exercise for strength and energy.
2. *Directional*—developing a joyful passion and noble purpose so a person might live a focused and self-motivating life in the pursuit of personal goals and fulfillment.
3. *Nutritional*—the need for good nutrients—food and beverages—that contribute to the healthy growth of new cells and the replacement of old ones.
4. *Emotional*—the need for establishing and building relationships marked by good communication, empathy, loyalty, and an ability to work together, laugh together, and cry together through a variety of circumstances and situations.
5. *Mental*—the "mental habits" that lead to positive words and beneficial deeds.
6. *Spiritual*—at the core of the five aspects of life above is the spiritual dimension of life. We each have a need for purity, faith, and forgiveness, and of establishing a beneficial and encouraging relationship with the Creator and other people.

The six aspects of the Totally Fit Life go together to make a star, with the spiritual at the core of the star. I call this the "Fitness Star."

I have always been in awe that it is the gravitational pull of the sun that keeps all of the planets in our solar system in perfect orbit and alignment. In the Fitness Star, it is the spiritual dimension of life that exerts "gravitational pull" to keep other aspects of life in balance and harmony. If the spiritual dimension of life is missing, weak, or unhealthy, other aspects of life invariably suffer—even if the person refuses to admit that they do!

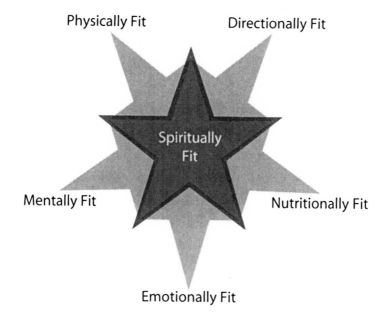

Physically Fit   Directionally Fit

Spiritually Fit

Mentally Fit   Nutritionally Fit

Emotionally Fit

Lucille and Ramona had a couple of questions—good ones. Ramona asked, "Why do you refer to these areas of life in terms of *fitness?*"

Answer: Technically speaking, to be fit means to be suitably adapted, adjusted, qualified, or capable for a specific purpose, function, or situation. In our case, as human beings, to be fit means to be in excellent condition as a whole human being to deal with the whole of human life!

Lucille wanted to know, "How can you tell if things are fit, or in balance?"

Answer: Life takes on a feeling of "wellness" or well-being. A person who is totally fit describes his or her life in terms such as *strong, solid, mature, vibrant, deep,* and *whole.* The six areas of life work together in a synergistic way, which is a five-dollar word for saying that the nature of the whole is far greater than just the sum of the various parts. There's a sense of being "in the groove" of your life's purpose. Perhaps most importantly from Lucille's standpoint, total fitness means *not* being able to pinpoint one area of life that is either *totally* missing or extremely lopsided.

Ramona also asked, "Aren't there other dimensions of life that contribute to total fitness?" I figured her recent divorce might be fueling that question, and I was right.

Certainly relationships are a big part of life, but relationships require the active will and participation of *two* people. You can't get fit on behalf of another person. What you can do is become as emotionally, mentally, and spiritually fit as possible, so that when you enter a relationship with someone, you have the best opportunity for establishing a good relationship.

Finances are also a big part of life, but financial solvency and material success aren't always dependent on what a person does. There are other factors at work—for example, employers who might decide to close a business; economic conditions in your city, state, or nation; market factors that may be related to your business sector; international and national political factors or wars; hurricanes that damage Gulf of Mexico oil rigs, and so forth.

You or your family may be hit with a serious accident or injury. You may have a spouse who overspends your family budget. You may suffer a theft or a natural disaster. The areas of fitness covered in this book are areas in which *you* have the sole or at least a highly significant share of the decision-making and choice-making responsibility and opportunity. You as an individual have the power to make key decisions about exercise, the life goals you set, eating patterns, emotional patterns you develop, your thought life, and the beliefs you hold.

Another person who asked a good question related to the Totally Fit Life was Daniel. He admitted to me that he had recently experienced a magical milestone birthday—sixty-one. I was a little surprised at that number and asked if he knew why that birthday had been such a threshold for him. He said, "My mom died just a month after she turned sixty-one. I think I've always thought that I might die at that age too."

He didn't. But for the next year, he *thought* he might! For twelve months I listened to Daniel ask, "Are you sure I'm not too old to be doing this?"

For twelve months I had to reassure him that I was not giving him an exercise plan, eating plan, goals, or any other "tool" related to the Totally Fit Life that was unsafe for him to do.

One day he asked, "Is a person *ever* too old to think about pursuing the Totally Fit Life?" The answer is no. There is no checkout age on the pursuit of health and well-being in any of the six areas of the Totally Fit Life. Certain physical conditions may make progress slower or more difficult toward greater-fitness goals, but very few conditions completely prohibit growth and improvement.

Start where you are. Take on the challenge. Do what you can do.

You will probably be pleasantly surprised at your own progress and success.

FOUR HALLMARKS OF TOTAL FITNESS

As you progress toward experiencing the Totally Fit Life, keep in mind the following four hallmarks. They are the greater goals, but they are also the descriptive words for the process of working toward greater fitness. Ask yourself from time to time, *Am I experiencing a life marked by greater* _____*?* Fill in the blank with one or more of the following words: *zest, growth, goodness,* and *choice.*

Zest
The Totally Fit Life is a life of great vibrancy and vitality. The person living a Totally Fit Life has a zest for life—a zest marked by strength and energy. As they age, many people begin to make statements such as, "I don't have the strength to do that anymore" or, "I don't have the energy

to do that." My response is always, "Well, what do you have the strength to do? What do you have the energy to do? Start there and seek to build strength and increase energy!"

Having sufficient strength and energy are key aspects of feeling well and whole. Begin with what you *can* do, and seek to build on that. It's only as you take steps to increase your strength and energy that you improve! If you don't have a deep feeling of vitality, accept the fact that you presently aren't enjoying a Totally Fit Life, and begin to explore ways in which you might come to have this life.

Growth

Life isn't static, and neither are life goals. The horizon shifts as we walk toward it, and that is true for fitness as well. The more fit we become, the more fit we *want* to be. Those who participate in the Totally Fit Life program tend to reach their initial goals and then set even higher goals. They begin to experience wholeness, and they want to be even more whole.

The Totally Fit Life program puts you on a path that doesn't end. But who cares if it does? You will be enjoying the journey so much that you won't be the least bothered that you still see areas where you want to grow, mature, progress, or scale higher heights.

There's no greater adventure than pursuing, achieving, and maintaining a Totally Fit Life. It's an exhilarating, exciting, enriching, and truly *enjoyable* way to live.

Goodness

I like the fact that the Creation story in the Bible tells us that God looked on every aspect of His creation and said, "It is good." The person who is living a Totally Fit Life has a life marked by goodness. He feels good. He eats good foods, drinks beverages that are good for him, and exercises in ways that are good for producing strength and energy. A person living a Totally Fit Life has good goals, thinks good thoughts, has good emotions, and builds good relationships. The Totally Fit Life is "wholesome"—it is a way of life that is *good* for a person!

Choice

If there's one thing I've discovered in visiting nursing homes and other retirement centers, it is that many of the residents in these facilities no longer make important choices regarding their own lives. They have given the responsibility of making choices and decisions to caregivers. The sad truth is that caregivers rarely make choices that compel a person to improve, grow, or become healthier or more fit. Caregivers generally make choices that allow a person to maintain. Maintenance is easier to manage for a caregiver than growth. Residents in these facilities are never encouraged to "make waves." But if you don't maintain, you decline.

If you don't make waves or create a wake, you're not moving. If you're not moving, you're dying.

Before the Totally Fit Life can be turned into a reality in your life, you must make a *choice* to embrace it, own it, and pursue it. A Totally Fit Life isn't an automatic gift to any person—it is something that requires choice and action.

Not long ago I heard about a woman who died from emphysema. She was a heavy smoker much of her life but hadn't smoked in twenty years. When she began to have breathing problems, her physician told her, "You need to enroll in some of the special exercise classes here at the hospital to increase your breathing ability."

This woman said to her husband on the way home from that appointment, with considerable agitation: "What does he think he's doing, telling me I need to go to exercise classes? I can hardly walk out to the car. I'll just be more tired if I go to those classes." She refused to go. Her lung health declined dramatically.

This woman made a *choice* about what she *would not do*.

She may not have understood one of the basic truths about exercise of all types: exercise is movement or activity that is designed to make a person stronger, not weaker. It is aimed at building up, not tearing down. This is true for all areas of the Fitness Star. If you want more physical energy and strength, you need to do physical exercise aimed at increasing your physical strength and energy level. If you want more emotional well-being, you need to do emotional exercise. Very often that involves taking the risk of reaching out beyond yourself to help others. If you want more spiritual fitness, generally you must exercise basic spiritual disciplines such as prayer, reading the Bible, and becoming involved in worship services. These disciplines are ones that help a person grow, mature, and become spiritually strong and vibrant.

The choices you make *will* determine the degree to which you become whole. They also determine to a great extent the degree and the rapidity of the aging process. What you choose *not* to do can directly impact how quickly you lose physical, mental, social, emotional, and spiritual capacity.

I routinely encounter people who think along these lines:

I've been fat so long that I can never be thin.
I'm too old now to change my ways.
I'll never be able to make a life change.
I've failed so many times I can't imagine that success is possible.
I'm so out of shape there's no hope for me.

None of the above are true. You may have come to the point where you sincerely believe these lies because you have repeated them so often. I'm here to tell you that these *are* lies and you *can* begin to believe the truth and start immediately to make the right choices and decisions that will put you on the path to a Totally Fit Life. The real question is: Do you want this? If you don't, there's *nothing* I can do. If you *do* want a Totally Fit Life, there are tremendous things I can do to help you!

What do you choose? Zest? Growth? Goodness? You may be just one choice away from having more of these qualities in your life.

Lucille and Ramona wanted greater fitness in their lives. At the end of my ten-week challenge to them, they signed up for another ten weeks, and then another. Three and a half years later, they are still walking together and they've taken on goals that they never dreamed of pursuing when they first began. Are they closer to living a Totally Fit Life today than they were thirteen hundred days ago? Definitely! Are they excited about the degree to which they have become fit? Absolutely! Do they still desire to be more fit? Assuredly.

The same is true for Steve and Tim and Craig and Mary Lou and Mark and Eugenia and Sam and hundreds of other people I could name. Those who choose to pursue a Totally Fit Life begin to experience that life, and part of the experience is invariably a greater zest for life, growth, and an abiding experience of "goodness" that they wouldn't trade for anything.

CHAPTER 3

The 5 Big Questions

Ben was forty-four years old when he said to me: "I thought I'd have more answers by now." I had known Ben for about five years, and I understood completely what he was saying. He had undergone treatment for malignant colon polyps and, although he had recovered fully and been cancer-free for more than three years, the specter of recurring cancer was there. Would he live out an average life span? He wondered.

Ben had pursued a career with great passion and energy and had enjoyed good success climbing the corporate ladder of his choosing. When the cancer appeared, he began to question if he was really doing what he wanted to do. He began to think in terms of legacy and leaving something worthwhile behind, and he wondered if his chosen career was really the right choice.

Ben put so much time and energy into his career in his twenties that the woman he married right after college walked out on him after only six years of marriage. He was devastated at the time but threw himself even more into his work. He had been dating a wonderful woman with two children for several years when he was diagnosed with cancer. Suddenly faced with his own mortality, Ben withdrew from the relationship.

The woman's heart was broken instantly, but Ben's heart seemed to break *after* his course of treatment was completed, which was several months down the line. He began to feel a deep loss, but he wondered if it was for this particular woman or if perhaps the feelings were ones that reflected a more generalized sense of loss because he didn't have a spouse and family. He wondered if it was too late to be a husband and perhaps even a father.

There were lots of questions in Ben's mind and heart. That is often the case for people after they turn forty, with or without a wake-up call of disease, accident, or tragedy. For many people, the questions seem to outnumber the answers.

There are five major questions that seem to occur with regularity as people cross the threshold of a magical milestone birthday. You may have asked these questions or perhaps have had a back-of-the-mind notion that you should address them. They *need* to be addressed if a person is truly going to enjoy a Totally Fit Life.

QUESTION #1: WILL I EVER FEEL YOUNG AGAIN?

This question tends to be asked in the wake of a physical setback, often after an accident or major ailment, but sometimes after a routine physical checkup or just over the course of life.

Maureen came to see me when she was forty-one. She had gone into early menopause—at the age of thirty-seven—and she tended to chalk up all of her problems to "the change." She felt *old*.

Some of Maureen's feelings were also rooted in the fact that she had just sent the younger of her two children off to college. She decided to go back to work as a means of coping with her empty nest. She applied for two jobs, and in each case a significantly younger person was hired. "Or at least they *looked* younger," Maureen said. One of the women hired was forty, but in Maureen's opinion she looked thirty. Maureen was discouraged.

So was Kate. In her case, she had been a schoolteacher for thirty years and at age fifty-four, she questioned how much longer she'd be able to keep up with her sixth graders. She needed to work to supplement the family income. She suffered, however, from chronic feelings of exhaustion and lower back pain.

Both Maureen and Kate asked, as Ben did in the aftermath of cancer treatment: "Can I ever feel young again?"

I pointed out to each of them that "young" was a term they needed to define. I gave them a questionnaire in which I asked them to mark the terms that they associated with feeling young. For most people, being young is associated with more laughter, more beauty, more freedom, more spontaneity, fewer aches and pains and less stiffness, and more energy. Let's break it down.

- *Laughter.* Joy is a choice. It is a matter of attitude and perspective, and as such, is totally unrelated to the number of calendar cycles you've experienced. I've met eighty-year-olds who still have a twinkle in their eyes and a chuckle on their lips.
- *Beauty.* There's a deep inner beauty that comes *only* with age. Again, beauty is rooted in attitude and perspective, not calendar years.
- *Freedom.* This is often equated with having fewer responsibilities and obligations. You may or may not be able to eliminate some obligations and commitments from your life, but you certainly can reevaluate the memberships you have, the care-giving that you do, and the commitments you have made involving time and finances. Adjustments are usually possible. But again, this is mostly a matter of making decisions and choices. Freedom is first and foremost an attitude.

- *Spontaneity.* No person should ever become so busy that he or she can't take one or two hours of downtime in any given day for reflection, recreation, and relaxation. Every person needs to have "margin" in his or her life, and margin is a concept that is related to both time management and attitude.

What I hope you will have noted about these four descriptive terms associated with youth is that they are rooted in how a person *thinks*. We'll cover this more in depth in a later chapter, but for now, recognize that there is an answer to the "Will I ever feel young again?" question, and the answer is that if you *think* young, you will *feel* young.

There are other defining characteristics of youth:

- *Fewer aches and pains, and less stiffness.* This is mostly a matter of flexibility, and flexibility is related to the degree a person stays in motion. *Keep moving!* That may mean continuing to work at tasks that require you to move. A woman told me that her mother had started to suffer from arthritic stiffness and pain in many of her joints. "But," the woman said, "not her fingers. The joints of her fingers began to look arthritic, but Mom had no pain or stiffness in them."

  "Why do you think that was?" I asked.

  "She kept typing!" was the immediate reply. "My mom used an old manual typewriter, and she could type 140 words a minute. She typed something every day. Even if it wasn't business related, she'd type a long letter to a grandchild or friend. Her rheumatologist told her that the finger and wrist action of typing was the greatest medicine he could prescribe for the arthritis in her hands."

  If the work you do doesn't require you to flex your muscles, then do flexibility-related exercises. There's more on this in a later chapter.

- *More energy.* Energy levels are directly related to nutrition and exercise—period. People feel sluggish and are exhausted *primarily* because they eat the wrong things, eat too much, or don't exercise. In some cases, a person may need supplements to restore good nutrition to the body at the cellular level. Back to the question, Will I ever feel young again? Part of the answer is that you probably can if you choose to exercise often and eat right.

What About Physical Ailments and Diseases?

About 80 percent of the degenerative diseases a person encounters with aging are diseases that can be reversed or greatly alleviated. There are a number of past health mistakes that you can undo.

Two of the biggest contributors to all forms of cardiovascular disease and autoimmune diseases, including cancer, are 1) smoking, and 2) poor nutrition, including obesity. A great deal of the suffering linked to cancer, heart disease, and other diseases commonly associated with aging can be eliminated if a person will stop smoking and start eating right—right foods, right beverages, in the right amounts. Smoking not only damages cells throughout the body, it also causes a person to look older. The same is true for obesity. In one study, people thought obese people were nine years older than they actually were!

So, can you feel young again?

Yes, if you want to—with your whole heart. The principles that are at the core of the Totally Fit Life program can help you feel—and look—younger.

QUESTION #2: IS MY LIFE
GOING TO MAKE A DIFFERENCE?

Only you can determine what gives you a sense of purpose, or what aspects of life are filled with the most meaning. Purpose and meaning are two important concepts for you to evaluate. They are especially important concepts to people after they have passed a magical milestone birthday.

Frank said to me one day, "Coach, I overheard what you said the other day to the woman who asked you why she was so listless and depressed. You were right."

I asked, "Have you ever felt that way?"

"Yeah, several years ago," Frank said. "I turned sixty-five a few years back and my company had a mandatory retirement policy. I enjoyed playing golf and working on a few things in my shop for a few months, but then I woke up one morning and said to the guy in my mirror, 'Frank, ol' buddy, nobody but your wife would care one bit if you went back to bed and didn't get up for two months.'"

"Wow," I said. "That was a pretty honest confrontation."

"It sure was," Frank said. "So, I decided I'd better get involved in something where people other than Helen *did* care if I showed up."

Frank went on to tell me that he became involved in building Habitat for Humanity houses. He was a skilled carpenter, and he also knew his way around electrical wires and plumbing problems. Frank became involved in building homes for low-income homeowners and, at the time we talked, he was on his fifteenth house!

He also started helping widows in his church with some of the repairs around their homes. Helen helped him with this, spending time talking or shopping with the women while Frank fixed air conditioning units and did household repairs.

"So people care now if you show up?" I asked. "And that makes a difference?"

"I have a *waiting list* of people who care," Frank laughed. He paused for a couple of moments and then he added: "Coach, I think I've helped more people in the last three years than in the previous thirty years. I know I've made a *good* difference in people's lives."

Part of knowing you've made a difference lies in *giving* to others. Part of making a difference is also related to a readjustment of priorities. For Evelyn, making a difference came when she made some changes in her priorities. She said to me, "Coach, when I turned forty-two, it suddenly hit me that both of my parents had died in their midsixties. I was two-thirds through my life if I lived as long as they did! That was a shocker."

"What did you do?" I asked.

"The first thing wasn't really related to priorities. It was related to the pace of my life. I didn't want to live the last third of my life—if that's all I had left before me—with so much stress. I faced up to the fact that I was going at a breakneck speed from the time I got up at six o'clock to the time I went to bed at midnight. I thought that in all my 'doing,' I was doing something worthwhile. The thought occurred that maybe everything I was doing wasn't necessary or important. I took a weekend away to evaluate my life. A few weeks before, I had gone to a special retreat in which the speaker suggested we make a list of everything we did in a week. So, I took that list, went to a beach house of a friend for a weekend, spread that list out in front of me, and really took a long, hard look at it."

"What did you learn?" I asked.

"I realized that I was spending about eight hours a day doing things that were of no earthly or heavenly benefit whatsoever. I had filled up hours with things that didn't really matter, so I started dropping some of those things. It was hard to say no at first, but it was tremendously freeing at the same time."

"That's a lot of time," I said.

"Six hours!" she said, apparently as surprised by what she had discovered as I was. "I added back into those hours about three hours of things that I felt were really important, and part of my reason for being on this earth. The other three hours I just used to do things a little more slowly, a little more carefully, and a little more thoroughly. The end result was really good—I got involved in a couple of things that made me feel as if I was really making a difference in the world. And I also started getting a lot more satisfaction in my work and other chores because I could see that I was doing things *well,* and not haphazardly."

From talking to a number of people through the years about meaning, purpose, and fulfillment, I've come to two major conclusions:

- Living *one* day with purpose can be more satisfying than living a decade without it. It isn't how *long* you have left to do something meaningful with your life; it's that you live *each day for the rest of your life with meaning.* It's never too late to start a new project or embark on a new venture that you find filled with purpose and meaning.
- Nobody but you can decide what gives you deep fulfillment. Don't let anybody else talk you into *their* "good cause." Take some time to explore what *you* have been uniquely gifted to do, what causes you to respond with an enthusiastic "Yes, let's!" attitude, and what makes the most of your specific skills, information, and personality.

Is it possible for you to still grab hold of a deep purpose for your life?
Is it possible for you to readjust your priorities?
Is it possible for you to infuse your daily activities with greater meaning?
Is it possible to live with less stress and more focus?
Absolutely! But only if you want to do what it takes to build greater meaning and purpose into your life. It comes down to directional choices. The Totally Fit Life includes directional fitness.

QUESTION #3: HAVE I REACHED
THE PINNACLE OF MY ABILITY?

Closely related to questions about the meaning and purpose of life are questions related to your progress in life and the ambition you feel—or don't feel—related to your progress.

A number of people who cross a magical milestone birthday begin to question the direction in which they are moving. Suspecting that perhaps they are climbing a ladder to success that is leading to a goal they don't really want, they slow down a little to reevaluate where they are going in life and why. I see this often in top-level corporate executives who discover at age sixty that they really don't *want* to be heading the corporation they are leading! They started up the ladder in their twenties and became so consumed by the thrills and challenges of the climb that they never stopped to evaluate if they were feeling fulfilled by their work. At the top of the ladder, they looked around and began to ask, *Is this all there is?* Too often the answer is no.

What generally follows is some sort of hiatus, retreat, sabbatical, or general withdrawal—sometimes for a few days, sometimes for a few weeks—while the person becomes introspective. Two things tend to happen as a result. First, there's a general loss of momentum. What was humming along at fast-lane speed suddenly slows. It's like a car that's been traveling in a straight line at 70 mph and, suddenly, the brakes are applied so the car can make a ninety-degree turn to the left or right, or perhaps even a U-turn.

Once the person has made a decision to move in a new direction, a second phenomenon kicks in. He finds that he feels less ambition toward the pursuit of the new direction or new goal. There seems to be a built-in reluctance to pursue the new goal too quickly, perhaps out of fear that this might not be the best or wisest choice. "I'll take it slow for a while and see if this is what I really want," Garth said to me one day.

Two months later I asked how he was enjoying his career change, and he said: "I think I like this. It feels right."

Another two months went by. I again asked how things were going, and Garth replied, "I'm a little concerned, Coach. I like what I'm doing, but I don't seem to have the ambition I had in my former career. When I was in my twenties and thirties I thought nothing of working sixty-hour weeks to get to the top of my game and to be the 'leader of the pack.' Now that I'm forty-eight, I resent working more than forty hours a week.

"In this new career, I'm enjoying the process more—you know, the day-to-day work—but I don't have any great goals. Earning enough to pay my bills and sock some away in an IRA seems to be all I care about. I'm wondering what happened to my ambition and if I'll ever get it back."

I talked to Garth at length that day, and here is a summary of the two main points we discussed. First, it seems that people who move from an unfulfilling career into one that they believe is or will be more satisfying, often move into a career that is "easier" for them. This may be a good thing. It may be that they are finally in the groove of what they are innately talented to do. They face less struggle in acquiring the skills necessary for successful performance.

In some cases, the person may be moving from work in a vocation to work in an area of avocation—perhaps a former hobby or interest has become a money-earning job or business for them. They know a lot about their hobby or interest, so they don't face a big learning curve. The tasks associated with the new career are already easy to do. They are already halfway up the new ladder, so they feel less urgency about the climb.

Second, those who move from an unfulfilling or unsatisfying career into a new career often find that they enjoy the new work much more than they enjoyed the old work. The tasks themselves are rewarding and pleasurable. They don't have any great desire to acquire more responsibility—especially supervisory responsibility—that may take them away from the task.

A woman said to me about her career, "I had four promotions in six years, each time to a higher position in the company that put me more and more in charge of telling other people what to do, rather than doing the work myself. One day I woke up and realized that I really missed the 'tasks' that I had been doing in my entry-level position. I didn't want to go back to the pay I got for doing those tasks, but I did want to have a job that was more hands-on and productive. I wanted less responsibility for other people."

What did this woman do? She quit her corporate job and started her own business. She supervised one person—herself. She did the tasks she was good at doing and enjoyed doing. She charged a reasonable amount for her services. And she led a much more fulfilling and satisfying life.

When I asked about her ambitions, she laughed and said: "I'm not as ambitious as I once was. I traded in ambition for happiness."

There's nothing about the Totally Fit Life that requires a person to be ambitious or to be in red-hot, super-intense, sharply focused pursuit of higher and higher goals. What the Totally Fit Life concepts do is to help people discover what types and levels of personal achievement would be fulfilling to them.

If a person is fulfilled at a job that has very little income—so be it.

If a person feels deep satisfaction in doing work that has very little fame associated with it—good for that person.

If a person has meaning and purpose for his or her life, even in doing something that has very little potential for international franchising—that's OK!

Not everyone is motivated by having lots of money, great fame, personal power, or widespread influence. What's important is to discover what you want in life and then have sufficient drive to reach it. And that's where we come to the flip side of this issue. There are some people who do *not* question the direction in which they are going. They like the direction of their lives, the career they are in, or the profession they chose. They still want to achieve the goals they set years ago for accomplishment in that chosen field of endeavor. They find themselves wondering, *Why am I not further along the road than I am toward the success I desire to have?*

Those people often became unfocused or scattered in their efforts—for any number of reasons. They may have become caught up in office politics or corporate downsizing or restructuring activities. They may have faced family or personal issues that sidetracked them from their overall purpose and goals. They may have become committed to activities, relationships, or organizations that drained them of time, energy, or resources—and, as a result, kept them from moving toward the fulfillment of their lives in a concerted, energetic way. Some people may have allowed themselves to become out of shape, overweight, easily exhausted, or overly stressed to the point that they simply no longer have the energy to sustain momentum toward goals they set.

Again, the Totally Fit Life principles call for you to reevaluate not only *where* you are headed but *how* you are pursuing your life goals and what might be impeding the accomplishment of those goals.

Finally, some people no longer have ambition, motivation, or drive, because they decided—consciously or subconsciously—that they know all that they need to know. They quit learning and, as a result, they quit growing. They moved over into the slow lane on the information highway, and other people who are acquiring more information and skills are passing them by. They need to make a decision to learn in order to grow.

All of these issues related to ambition and reaching the pinnacle of one's ability are addressed in the Totally Fit Life. There's nothing about the aging process that inherently squelches ambition.

A friend told me about one of his mentors, a tremendously talented man who was a stage designer for television, movies, and the theater. This designer—now ninety years old—was still going to work four days a week, working six hours a day, and in the opinion of my friend, was at the top of his game when it came to design. Furthermore, this ninety-year-old designer was still driving to work!

"What fuels his passion?" I asked.

"He doesn't think he's come up with his best design yet," my friend said. "He still believes that tomorrow a new job might come in that will challenge him to do the best work of his life."

That's the underlying attitude necessary for a person to achieve a Totally

Fit Life—regardless of age. Ambition, motivation, and drive ultimately come down to a person pursuing the work of his choosing with the idea: *There's still one more thing I can do, should do, or want to do—and do it better than I've ever done anything before.*

QUESTION #4: IS THIS ALL THE HAPPINESS I CAN EVER HOPE TO HAVE?

Midlife seems to be a time when people begin to reevaluate their relationships with great intensity. Many people look deep within and question, *Shouldn't I be happier?*

Perhaps people in all cultures feel they have a right to be happy, but I have a hunch that especially in our culture people feel that happiness is a birthright. Everywhere around me in our society I see people who are willing to trade in long-standing commitments so they can pursue a rather fleeting feeling of happiness. People frequently tell me they are making certain changes in their lives because "I'm just not happy with the ways things are" or "I think I'll be happier if I make this change."

Linda gave me the happiness argument as her justification for leaving her husband of twenty-eight years. "He just didn't make me happy," she said. Then she realized what she had said and added, "I probably didn't make him happy." I listened and didn't respond. She decided to edit her statement one more time: "Actually, neither one of us was happy any longer."

"How long ago did you leave your husband?" I asked.

"Two years ago," she said.

"Are you happier?" I asked.

"Oh yes!" she said.

"In what ways?" I asked.

Linda spent the next five minutes telling me all the things she could do now that she couldn't have done when she was married.

"Let me get this straight," I said. "You *couldn't* do those things when you were married or you just *didn't* do them?"

She paused. "I guess I didn't know I could do them," she finally said.

"Is there anything you miss about being married?" I asked.

She cried for the next half hour. I hadn't meant to break through the shell around such a reservoir of tears, but I did. The best I could do to comfort Linda was to sit in silence next to her as she cried. In the end, Linda admitted she *wasn't* happier since she ended her marriage. She was forty-four years old and she had managed to take all the unhappiness of her marriage with her into her new single life—leaving behind some things that now seemed valuable to her. Linda had pursued personal happiness, without really understanding that happiness is rarely achieved in pursuing something that is focused on *self*.

The pursuit of happiness seems to be rather common among forty-something, even fifty-something and sixty-something people who don't feel loved or aren't satisfied in their marriages. A few people with whom I've had intense conversations feel almost desperate to experience what seems to have eluded them thus far in their lives. For some reason, they never seem to have addressed the idea that real happiness is found in *giving*, not in receiving.

Midlife also seems to be a time when people who have a strained or unsatisfying relationship with their children seek to reach out in new ways. Others seem suddenly in midlife to have a deep desire to establish and build a good relationship with their grandchildren—bypassing the miserable relationship they have with their own children. In each of these situations, the people seem to be looking for a level of emotional pleasure that they haven't experienced previously. They often are very candid in stating that they are not emotionally fit, and they generally equate that lack of emotional fitness to a mystical happiness gauge.

The Totally Fit Life is not lived in pursuit of happiness—primarily because happiness is a fleeting emotion that is dependent for the most part upon outward circumstances or situations. Happiness ebbs and flows. It is nearly always directly linked to the immediate environment in which a person finds himself. What is lasting and of much great benefit is *joy*. The Totally Fit Life is marked by genuine joy.

Joy comes when a person takes *delight* in the world around him, refuses to live in anxiety or high stress, and recognizes that life is filled with foibles, eccentricities, and antics. Joy is the atmosphere in which most children dwell—at least those who are healthy and live in abuse-free environments. To have greater joy, think like a child! Pause to consider all of the ordinary miracles in any given day—from the unique patterns of fingerprint design on the tips of your own fingers to the brilliant sunset in the western sky. Reactivate your own curiosity. Explore. Regain a sense of wonderment at the world.

Watch and allow yourself to be amused by the antics of children and animals, especially baby animals. If you have totally lost your sense of humor, start with smiling. Choose to smile at the way the sun hits the autumn-colored leaves outside your window, the way the neighbor's puppy chases the first snowflakes it has ever seen, and the surprised look that comes across your friend's face when she realizes she has *not* said what she *thought* she said. Life has funny moments that should be appreciated as funny!

Joy comes when a person expresses thanksgiving and appreciation. Joy comes when a person praises others and acknowledges the good deeds or accomplishments of others. Joy comes when a person praises and thanks God.

The joyful person looks outward from a depth of inner joy and asks: *What can I do to help others or give to others?* The happiness-seeking person looks inward from a lack of happiness and asks: *Why aren't people doing more to make me happy?*

The joyful person does not seek to be the center of the universe, but, rather, seeks to help create a better home life, church life, or community life for everyone involved.

In my opinion, the best response to the question, Is this all the happiness I can ever hope to have? is to say: "You're asking the wrong question. The right question to ask is, Can I experience an abiding joy deep within my soul?" The answer to this second question is yes, and the Totally Fit Life principles can help a person experience that type of joy. Joy is a key part of emotional fitness.

QUESTION #5: WHAT WILL HAPPEN AFTER I DIE?

The question at the core of spiritual fitness is one of the key questions of the ages: What happens after death? This is a question that midlife people nearly always begin to ask with renewed intensity and concern. Very often the question comes in the wake of a parent's funeral, or after both parents have died. A person suddenly finds himself at the top of the family tree, staring straight up into the heavens with no people in between who "should die first."

At other times, a major illness or the threat of one can cause a person to confront his or her mortality. Ben, the man I mentioned at the outset of this chapter, admitted to me that he had spent many hours on his knees in prayer preparing himself spiritually for the "probability I might die."

He said, "Coach, after the chemotherapy doc told me all I was facing, I went home and sat down on my sofa and said out loud, 'I could die.' It suddenly hit me that death was not a matter of could or could not. The truth is, I *will* die, maybe not from colon cancer, but certainly some day I'm going to die from something. I decided right then and there I needed to settle the death issue. I needed to decide once and for all that I was prepared to die."

"That put you at peace?" I asked.

"Absolutely," Ben said. "But it did something more than that, Coach."

"What?" I asked.

"When I settled the death issue, I also settled the life issue," Ben said. "When I knew I was prepared to die, I also knew I was fully prepared to live. The things that were important for me to get straight and to have as priorities before I died were the things I needed to *keep* straight and *keep* as priorities every day from now until I die. I had a new focus and freedom for *living*. I still have lots of questions, but when it comes to the biggest question, I have an answer. I know where I'm going when I die."

He's 100 percent on target. Dying is not a matter of *if*. It's a matter of *when*. There are some things that *should* be faced before death, and they tend to be the most important things of life. I asked Ben what he considered to be the foremost issues associated with dying. He cited these five: 1) dying with a deep sense of peace that everything was right with his Creator; 2) knowing God and other people had forgiven him, and that he had forgiven everybody he needed to forgive; 3) having loving relationships—giving love and being open to receiving love; 4) having faith that God was in control of his life and that God was waiting for him in eternity; and 5) having a strong hope about heaven and the good things that were still to come.

Those who come to grips with the foremost death issues also come face-to-face with the key ingredients of a spiritually fit life:

- Peace with God
- Forgiveness—being forgiven, and freely forgiving
- Love—expressed in healthy give-and-receive relationships
- Faith
- Hope

The Totally Fit person has spiritual fitness at the core of his or her being—it is the area of fitness that impacts all other areas of life. You can't live a whole, harmonious, peace-filled life without having spiritual peace. You can't be emotionally whole without a flow of forgiveness and love in your life. You won't seek to accomplish any of the goals associated with total fitness unless you *believe* you can achieve them—and have faith that you *will* achieve them—with God's help. You won't have genuine directional or attitudinal fitness unless you have hope that the best is yet to be.

Seek spiritual fitness as your top priority. It's the fitness that has the greatest impact on eternity.

COACH'S CLIPBOARD

I'm a coach, and coaches give their players specific exercises as a part of workout drills. So . . . here are your exercises for this chapter!

Do you feel as young as you want to feel?

Exercise: Make a list of several of the traits that you associate with the word *young.* After you write each trait, reflect on it and next to it write two or three things you will do to add *more* of that trait to your life.

Is your life making a difference?

Exercise: Reflect about the kind of difference you'd *like* to make. Write down your thoughts and ideas here.

Have you reached the pinnacle of your ability?

Exercise: What additional skills or knowledge do you need to reach the top? List several.

Do you have joy?

Exercise: Identify two or three very practical things you might do to add more joy to your life. Take a moment to make note of those things here.

Have you settled the "after death" question?

Exercise: This is the most important question you'll ever answer. Take the time to think seriously about it, and commit now to coming to the answer YES.

TOTALLY FIT LIFE TRUTH

Getting the right answers is a matter of asking the
right questions and answering them honestly.

CHAPTER 4

Making Changes and Making the Changes Work

I'm a "how" person. Most of the time I don't deal in a lot of theory or pie-in-the-sky ideas. I am a coach. I deal in the practical and tactile issues of life: What do we *do* to win the game? What drills do we run? What routines do we establish? How do we *live* in a way that ensures we are going to show up on game day as prepared as possible for the biggest win attainable?

You may think I'm talking about some type of sport. I'm talking about *life*. Greater health and wholeness don't just happen—they must be *made* to happen. Achieving the Totally Fit Life requires change and growth, and change and growth require effort.

One of the first questions I ask when I read a book that contains good information about how to live a healthier or more fit life is: *What makes this work?* The Totally Fit Life program is not just a set of concepts or principles. It is also a methodology—a way of responding to life that helps a person put the concepts and principles into practice.

There are three keys that make the Totally Fit Life program work for a lifetime and not just for a day. They are the keys that keep this way of living from being a fad and make it an ongoing life journey. They are keys that are timeless. They work for thirty-year-olds and seventy-year-olds. The keys are: frame goals in a ten-week cycle, become part of a Team of 3®, and speak dictums to yourself daily.

KEY #1: TEN-WEEK CYCLES

I don't know too many people who like hearing the phrases, "You can never again . . ." or "You have to do this the rest of your life." Change at that level is daunting.

"Do you think you can do this for two weeks?" That is the question I usually ask people who come to me desiring to implement the Totally Fit Life program. Nobody has ever said no to that question. When I ask, "Do you think you can do this for ten weeks?" most people say, "I think so." Some people may have a few doubts, but generally speaking, they are willing to give the program a try for ten weeks. Beyond that, commitment gets iffy.

The Totally Fit Life calls on you to set goals for yourself on a ten-week cycle. Every ten weeks you also have the opportunity to revise your Team of 3® and the dictums you speak to yourself daily. You may add to, delete from, or keep the regimen you have been pursuing. Regardless of your choice, you will be asked to make an intentional, written *new* commitment to pursuing your goals for ten weeks.

There are five main aspects I want to address related to the ten-week cycle: motivation, priorities, revisions, habit building, and ongoing cycles.

Motivation

Recently a woman said to me, "I love three holidays—New Year's Day, Memorial Day, and Labor Day." I thought that was a rather odd choice of days, so I asked why.

She said, "They are do-over days. On New Year's Day I can start new goals for a new calendar year. On Memorial Day I can start goals specifically for the summer ahead. On Labor Day, I can start 'school year' goals, even though I haven't been in school for years."

These would not have been my three choices for days of new beginning, but I do understand the motivation that comes from having a set time to start something. Many people would never dream of starting a diet on a Thursday—it's always "next Monday." Some business people tend to think in terms of quarterly goals for their personal lives as well as their professional lives. They wouldn't dream of starting a new program forty-one days into a quarter.

There's a surge of motivation anytime a person adopts or readopts a goal. A ten-week cycle will give you a fresh start time to gear up again, make a renewed commitment, climb back on the wagon, or give your goal another shot!

Priorities

A ten-week cycle also gives a person a good opportunity to see if a goal is really a priority goal—something that *must* be done if life is to be truly fulfilling. Periodically we each need to step back and reevaluate our use of time, resources, and the commitments we make.

Every ten weeks is a good time to give yourself a half hour of alone time to take an objective look at what you've done and not done, reflect upon why you may have failed in some areas, and to renew your commitment to those things that you see as an integral part of your ongoing success and growth.

Revisions

In the sections that follow we'll be discussing the concepts I call Team of 3® and Speaking Dictums. A Team of 3® relationship may be uncomfortable for a number of reasons. You may feel left out by the other two partners. You may not want to keep pursuing specific goals that the other two team members want to pursue. You may have met new people with whom you seem to be in better sync. The ten-week cycle allows you to make adjustments in the Team of 3® without long excuses, hurt feelings, or tearful partings.

You may also find after ten weeks of speaking dictums to yourself that you want to make adjustments in those dictums. Ten weeks is a good time for appraisal. You can be confident that you've given the old dictums a good hearing, and either benefited from them a little, a lot, or somewhere in between.

Habit Building

A ten-week period is a good length of time for establishing a new habit or breaking an old one. Behavioral modification experts have long held to the opinion that it takes at least this long for a mature adult to imprint a new habit. This applies to both mental and physical habits.

It takes ten weeks to see changes in your body as the result of daily exercise.

It takes ten weeks to adjust your eating so you no longer have intense cravings.

It takes ten weeks to cleanse the body of certain toxins and to renew the body's ability to taste certain foods (without an overlay of too much sugar, fat, or chemical preservatives).

It takes ten weeks to imprint a new idea on the mind.

Give yourself ample time for the *good* aspects of the Totally Fit Life to take hold and start reaping rewards.

Ongoing Cycles

The ideal, of course, is for you to choose to renew your goals, keep the same Team of 3®, and keep speaking daily dictums that move you forward on the path you've chosen to walk. Those who "re-up" for a second ten weeks very often find it much easier to re-up for a third ten-week cycle. By then they are starting to see real changes and to establish a deeper relationship with their team partners.

A significant change happens to those who re-up for a fourth cycle and complete it. I don't know why this is so, but I know from years of experience that there's something truly transformative about the forty-week mark. It is at this point that a habit seems to be established. Emotions often take this long to be fully healed or mental thought patterns to be changed. It often takes this long for a person to work through grief or the sorrow following a divorce.

Forty weeks is a time when many people find themselves feeling a renewed energy or sense of well-being from a major surgery, illness, or injury. I've also noted through the years that at the end of the fortieth week, many people report a strong sense of progress. They see a pattern of growth and change that is rewarding.

Also after four cycles, an individual often concludes, *Just one more cycle and I will have done this for a year!* Those who have been faithful to a program for forty weeks seem to see an imaginary finish line looming before them, and they are almost eager to accomplish an entire year of discipline, growth, and accountability. Once a year is over, it's not at all uncommon for a person to think, *I'm taking on another year. I'm on a roll!*

"But," you may be saying, "five cycles of ten weeks only adds up to fifty weeks, Coach. There are fifty-two weeks in a year. What about the other two weeks?"

Take them as a vacation! You may want a full two weeks off, or a few days off between each cycle.

I also strongly encourage you to take off one day a week as a "free" day. Call it a Sabbath day if you want. Call it a break day. That's a day when you will *not* need to check in with your Team of 3® partners, speak dictums, or log your activities or chart your progress. Consider this day a pause that refreshes. Use it as a time for reflections or for a renewal of commitment to your goals.

KEY #2: TEAM OF 3®

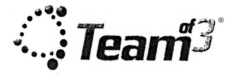

When I first explained the Team of 3® concept to Kay, she said, "I already have a walking partner."

"Is she an accountability partner?" I asked.

Kay paused for a few moments and then said, "In a way."

"What does that mean?" I asked.

"Well, she knows if I walk or don't walk on any given day, and she usually knows the reason why I can't walk with her."

"How many times in a month do you call each other to say that one of you *can't* walk on that day?" I asked.

"Oh, probably seven or eight times," she said.

"And you're walking four times a week?" I asked.

"Yes, that's our plan," she said.

"If you don't walk seven or eight times in a month, that's almost two weeks worth of walking!"

Kay was getting a little uncomfortable. "I can see where you're going," she said. "And you're right. The truth is, Martha and I aren't all that good for each other. It doesn't take much for one of us to say, 'Let's go get breakfast' as we head out for our walk. We end up at a cafe nearby and never do make it to the track."

I certainly had no intention of limiting the friendship that Martha and Kay had developed over years of their exercising together. Both were widows in their late sixties and they enjoyed their times together several days a week. What I did suggest was that they each become part of a new Team of 3® for real accountability purposes. Furthermore, I suggested that they be on separate teams. We found two team partners for Kay and

45

two for Martha. That way they could maintain the closeness of their friendship without feeling as if they had taken on an interloper.

When three people share a common set of goals, they *each* are much more likely to achieve their personal goals. That's the foremost reason for being part of a Team of 3® (see our Web site: www.teamof3.com).

How Does a Team of 3® Work?

In a Team of 3®, three people bind themselves together in a verbal agreement to pursue the Totally Fit Life. There are no contracts and nothing legally binding. It is a person-to-person agreement. Each person is saying to the other two, "I want to become totally fit. I'm willing to give you encouragement to help you become more fit, and I'm willing to receive your encouragement in return. Let's do this together."

Each team needs a leader. This is the person who is willing to say to the other two, "Let's meet at this time in this location," or call the group to greater accountability, saying, "Hey, team, we aren't living up to what we agreed to do. Let's renew our commitment."

Team of 3® members do these things for one another: define their own relationship and set their own goals, stay in daily contact, serve as accountability partners—reporting their progress toward goals—and encourage one another.

Defining Your Team Relationship

Henry was something of a loner. He left a corporate engineering job to establish his own highly specialized engineering company, which was a successful but stressful venture. The only other people involved in the company were his wife, who kept the books, and his two sons, one of whom was a computer expert and the other a civil engineer. Hank wasn't very communicative, and he wasn't much interested in being accountable to anybody. "Why do I need a team?" he asked. "I can just do this on my own."

"It's possible," I said. "Just not probable."

Henry knew that he needed to make some changes in his life, and he had a desire to pursue the Totally Fit Life program. He had experienced a heart problem that involved insertion of two stents into his cardiovascular system. His family and clients were depending upon his recovery, and he personally desired to live a more balanced and whole life. He was motivated and committed. The question is always, For how long?

Some people can muster up self-motivation and make it last for several weeks. Fewer are able to self-sustain their own motivation for several months. Most people are incapable of self-sustaining maximum motivation toward goals longer than a year or two.

"I'm not much of a team player," Henry admitted. "I have a very specialized business—and I think I like having a specialized life."

I explained to Henry that his personal goals for living the Totally Fit Life would also be highly specialized. "Nobody has precisely your set of desires, dreams, talents, brainpower, commitments, or responsibilities," I said. "Everything about you is unique, Henry, and I'm not here to take away from your individuality in the least. The Team of 3® exists to help you achieve your maximum *personal* best. The other two people are like cheerleaders and tax accountants at the same time. They exist to cheer you on to win *your* race and to keep your losses to a minimum while keeping all of your assets strong.

"Ultimately the goals you have for the Totally Fit Life are personal goals—nobody is going to mirror exactly the physical, directional, emotional, nutritional, mental, or spiritual goals that you desire to adopt. Even if your goals are similar to those of another person, your starting place and ending place may be very different. For example, you and another person may both desire to lose weight, but you may have fifty pounds to lose and the other person only fifteen pounds. You and another person may both desire to lower your cholesterol count by fifty points, but you may be starting with a cholesterol count of 200 and the other person may be at 250.

"You and another person may both desire to develop a deeper relationship with God, but you may sense that your need is to grow in your understanding of God as a faithful provider, while the other person may desire to grow in his understanding of God as a loving father. Where you will benefit most from having two other people as your team members are in the areas of motivation, accountability, and encouragement."

I said to Henry, "Don't you find that you do some things in your business on any given day because your sons are counting on you to finish your part of a project, or your wife is expecting you to have enough billable hours at the end of the week to ensure that your income will be sufficient?"

"Sure," he said.

"That's the reason for a Team of 3®," I said. "You'll find it much easier to stay on track as you pursue your goals if you have two people who are expecting you to help them and who are counting on you to do your part."

I recognized that Henry had some communication limitations. He wasn't a man who revealed much about what he was thinking or feeling. I asked, "Are you afraid this might become some kind of counseling or therapy group?"

"Correct," Henry replied in a very "engineering" tone of voice.

"This isn't about counseling," I said. "A Team of 3® is a *task*-oriented group. Team of 3® members share information and encourage one another on the specifics that are related to tasks—how you eat, what you do, how much you exercise, and in general, other data that indicates whether you are making progress toward a goal."

The degree to which you share information with your team members is up to you. You don't need to tell another person any specifics that you don't want to tell! You don't need to tell how much you weigh, the details of your marriage problems, the nature of the problems you are having at work, or the reason you want to change or improve in a specific area of your life. You don't need to admit any faults, flaws, or failures. You don't need to reveal any feelings or give any opinions. The reporting to your team members is rooted in *fact*.

What is required is a willingness to say to your two partners, "I want to improve. I would like your encouragement. I would like for you to hold my feet to the fire a little without nagging me."

Being accountable to two other people is the strongest motivator I've found in more than twenty years of life coaching. Being part of a Team of 3® is a potent force for compelling you to actually *do* what it is that you know or believe you should do.

Choosing Team of 3® Members

The ideal Team of 3® links three people who have something in common. Sometimes team members work for the same company, attend the same church, live in the same neighborhood, are about the same age, have children in the same college, or are recovering from the same disease. When team members have something in common, there's greater empathy for the successes and failures of the other partners, and also a greater understanding of the temptations that can pull a person off track.

A woman told me that she didn't initially feel she had much in common with her other Team of 3® members, but the four things they did have in common were more than sufficient for motivation and encouragement purposes. All three of them loved chocolate, they were in their late forties, they were morning people, and each woman was seeking the Totally Fit Life not only for long-range purposes but for a short-range goal of a thirty-year high school reunion! These three women happened to live in different states—they were linked up together through our Internet site—but they had strong nutritional and physical fitness goals. They were great together as a team. (Again, our site is www.teamof3.com.)

Miriam said, "If June or Alice told me that they had *not* met their nutritional goals for a given day, I knew they had probably given in to a chocolate urge. Nine times out of ten I was right. The three of us began to find little tidbits of information about chocolate to share with one another."

"Like what?" I asked.

"Like the fact that a person has to walk a hundred yards just to work off the calories of a single M&M."

"That was motivating?" I asked.

"It was to us!" Miriam said. "Especially when you also know that you are each trying to get into a smaller dress size."

These women communicated by e-mail at seven o'clock each morning, after they had exercised and before they headed for work or got busy with home chores. "If one of us hadn't exercised by then, we knew we needed to give that partner *extra* encouragement because as a morning person, if she didn't exercise before getting caught up in her day, we knew she'd have no energy or desire to exercise in the late afternoon or evening."

"Did you do anything else to help one another?" I asked.

"We sent each other songs," she said. "We'd download onto our computers songs that were popular when we were in high school. Since we are all pretty much the same age, we had all danced to the same music. We'd find funny things to say about the songs, and since they were high school songs, they all tied in some way to our upcoming reunions."

"Did you make your goals?" I asked.

"Yes!" Miriam reported with obvious joy in her voice. "We were twenty-two weeks away from the first reunion on the calendar when we started working together as a Team of 3® and twenty-nine weeks away from the third reunion. We each met our goals. Alice was a little bit of an overachiever. She lost more weight than June or me.

"We were each so pleased with our progress and the results that at the end of the summer we decided to re-up for a fourth ten-week cycle, and then a fifth. We're now into our second year of encouraging one another as a Team of 3®, and we're planning to celebrate our second full anniversary of teamwork by having a team meeting in about six weeks. We are going to meet together at a spa. It will be the first time we've seen each other face-to-face, but in many ways, I feel as if I'm about to go on vacation with old friends."

In choosing your Team of 3® partners I strongly recommend that you partner-up with people of your same sex. Because friendships are likely to emerge, and sometimes it is easy for a friendship to slip over the lines of marital fidelity, I believe people should stick to all-male or all-female teams. There are several other things you need to guard against.

First, guard against pairing off and leaving the third person alone. Don't exclude one team member or favor one more than another. Second, avoid feeling as if you must become "pen pals" with your team members. You certainly *may* choose to tell your team members why you are struggling in a certain area, but don't put other team members into a position in which they feel they have to respond as an empathetic counselor. Brief, one-sentence or two-sentence messages that are more factual than confessional are better. Keep your communication short and simple.

Third, don't compete against one another. Your team members are part of *your* team—cooperate, don't compete. Now, this isn't to say that you might not get involved in a great team competition against other Team of 3® groups. We've helped a number of companies, churches, gyms, and clubs establish competitions aimed at improving the overall fitness level of the larger group. Teams may compete against one another; individuals should not.

Competitions Among Teams

If you do decide to set up a competition with another team, make sure the rewards (some call them incentives) are ones that are helpful and healthful. I've seen various things offered as rewards that are completely appropriate for the Totally Fit Life, including a piece of exercise equipment named in honor of a team in the new church fitness center, a blender for making healthful fruit smoothies donated to a company kitchen, concert tickets, magazine subscriptions, and tickets to a baseball game. One company offered one prize for the winning female team and another for the winning male team. The women competed for a day at a spa and the men for tickets to a fishing tournament.

Daily Reporting of Activities

The main function of a Team of 3® is to have team members report to one another their participation in activities that are directly related to their goals. We use a very simple reporting system on our Internet site. You can use that system or develop one of your own. Be sure to keep the reporting system simple—one that you can use as a checklist without additional words, or the need to provide details. Here's our basic checklist (more about TOP 1™ later):

Eating:	☐ good	☐ fair	☐ poor
Activity:	☐ good	☐ fair	☐ none
Attitude:	☐ good	☐ fair	☐ poor
TOP 1™:		☐ yes	☐ no
Quiet time:		☐ yes	☐ no

You may want to add other specialized categories for your particular group; it's possible to customize this on our Web site. Henry, as a person recovering from heart-related surgery, was teamed up with two people who also had undergone stent procedures. His Team of 3® added this line to their daily report:

Took all meds:	☐ yes	☐ no

On one occasion I worked with a church that was focused on marriage enrichment. The teams that formed out of that group added these lines to their daily reporting:

Hugged and kissed spouse:	☐ yes	☐ no
Told spouse "I love you":	☐ yes	☐ no
Encouraged spouse:	☐ yes	☐ no

Does such a direct and objective means of reporting eliminate all opportunity for team members to write additional comments? Not at all. On the other hand, teams of engineer types such as Henry would balk at any suggestion that they *had* to write additional comments. All narrative reports should be totally optional, and at the discretion of the group. I recommend adding a place in a reporting form for a quick narrative line or two if a person wants to write a comment.

Here are some examples of a few ideal narrative comments:

Jerilyn: "I read my Bible today and had a prayer time, but not as long as I usually do. I felt guilty about that. At least I ate good and exercised. I know I really need to work on better balance."

Yvette: "I had really good insights today into *why* I can't seem to stay out of the fast-food drive-through lanes. One thing I've done is change the route I take to get home."

Tim: "Lousy attitude by the end of the day. I chalk it up to doing no exercise before work and then pigging out at lunch. Heading for a quiet time—maybe that will help me end the day on a good note."

How long does it take to check items on the basic checklist? About ten seconds.

How long does it take to add a couple lines of narrative if you choose to do so? About thirty seconds. In all, "reporting in" to your other team members can and *should* take less than a minute a day. (The Team of 3® Web site has a built-in easy means to send e-mail to teammates.)

Focus on Encouragement

I don't have any doubt that you can guess how the team partners of the three people above responded to their brief narrative comments.

Jerilyn's partners said to her: "Forgive yourself" and "I believe you'll do better tomorrow. Balance is tough."

Yvette's partners wrote back: "Good idea!" and "I'm going to try that."

Tim's partners responded: "I often pig out at lunch if I haven't exercised" and "I'm guessing the quiet time turned things around and you'll have a perfect report tomorrow."

It took these team members less than thirty seconds each to read and respond to the narrative comments noted above. Did the team members who received these messages find them helpful? Absolutely. Jerilyn felt forgiven and encouraged, Yvette felt affirmed and helpful, and Tim felt uplifted and motivated to get up and exercise the following morning.

KEY #3: SPEAK DAILY DICTUMS

The Totally Fit Life program certainly does not give your Team of 3® partners the license to nag you. Their role is encouragement. The program *does* encourage you to learn to nag yourself—but even in nagging yourself, I encourage you to do it in an *encouraging* way.

Rather than riding yourself for being stupid, lazy, out of shape, or lacking in willpower, try inner messages such as, *You're smarter than that, You can do this, You have what it takes,* and *You're getting better.* Be honest— you'd enjoy hearing those comments from someone you love. Learn to love yourself a little more and you'll enjoy hearing those comments from yourself!

Not long ago Annie said, "You know, Coach, what you said about learning to like fresh fruits and vegetables is what my mother says to me at least once a day."

"Really?" I asked. "Does your mother live with you?" I have many midlife acquaintances who are in their forties and fifties and have their elderly parents living with them.

"No," Annie laughed. "My mother lives in heaven!"

"But you said—" I started in.

She quickly cut me off. "Coach, it doesn't matter in the least that Mom died seven years ago. I can hear her voice in my head as crystal clear as if she were standing two feet away!"

Annie wasn't into mystical or paranormal experiences. She just had a very strong "tape player" in her mind that seemed to specialize in playing old messages recorded by her mother.

"Have you ever thought about replacing your mother's voice with your own voice?" I asked.

For the next few weeks, I worked with Annie to teach her how to establish daily dictums for herself—dictums that were directly related to her personal goals. She later reported to me, "I haven't heard from Mom in a long time now—at least not in a nagging way. I listen to myself and you know, Coach, I pay a lot more attention to me than to Mom."

That's true for most people. Nobody can command you like *you*. Call it self-motivation. Call it giving yourself a mental kick into gear. Call it whatever you like—just do it.

What's a Dictum?

A dictum is a command statement. It is a formal, authoritative pronouncement that you make to yourself—speaking the statement *aloud*. A dictum is a firm commitment, rooted in a conviction, that what you are pronouncing is going to happen.

It is totally up to *you* to decide the habits you want to develop, the changes you want to make, the practices you want to adopt, and as a result, the daily tasks that you want to pursue. Therefore, it is totally up to *you* to decide the dictums that you speak to yourself.

There's a basic progression that occurs between the things you *do* and the person you *become*. The formula is this:

Repeated behaviors ... become habits

and

Repeated habits ... become character

Your character is ultimately the sum of your repeated behaviors that have become habits. Every behavior has the ability to impact character.

Dictums are commands about who you *are* and what you will *do*. They are not pie-in-the-sky or future oriented. They are practical, specific, and possible to do and be *right now.*

"*I will*" dictums are specifically related to behavior and we cover these more in the Mental Fitness chapter. Here are examples of three "*I will*" dictums:

- I WILL spend time in prayer.
- I WILL eat good and healthful food.
- I WILL exercise.

I am statements are dictums specifically related to your character. Here are examples of three "*I am*" dictums:

- I AM a person of fervent prayer.
- I AM a person fueled by good nutrition.
- I AM strong, flexible, and energetic.

Over time, and the more you speak dictums, the more you are likely to gravitate to speaking only "*I am*" dictums. The reason some people cannot start out at that place is because they feel they are lying to themselves. They don't yet have a full vision for who they can be and are on their way to becoming. Once a person sees that he or she is moving into the character traits and identity he or she wants to have, the person usually feels much freer to speak "*I am*" dictums with great enthusiasm. "*I am*" dictums have much higher potency than "*I will*" dictums.

Commanding Your Priority Goals into Being

In all areas of the Totally Fit Life, you will be encouraged to become fit, not just *do* fitness-type things. There's a huge difference. Let me give you an example.

Art came to me and said after he had heard a full explanation of the Totally Fit Life: "I guess I have to walk."

"You guess?" I asked.

"OK," he said with a little more strength to his voice. "I *have* to walk."

"What's the dictum for that, Art?" I asked.

"OK," he said. "I *will* walk *today*."

"And in three weeks what do I want you to be saying to yourself as a dictum each morning?"

It took him a moment, but with great strength in his voice, Art finally said, "I *am* a fit, energetic, rapid-stepping walker."

"When?" I asked.

"OK!" Art nearly shouted at me. "I *am* a fit, energetic, rapid-stepping walker *today!*"

Art got it! The amazing thing was that I had not told Art to increase his volume or the strength of his voice the closer he came to giving me a true "*I am*" dictum. That happened naturally. It happens on the inside of a person, too. To see yourself as a "walker" is to see yourself in a positive position of strength. It's seeing yourself as a person with inner substance, discipline, and endurance. Those are character traits. To say "I am" about yourself, even if you haven't been walking regularly for very long and even if you haven't started on a walking routine, is to speak something about who you know you are on the *inside*.

The inside you is just waiting to be manifested on the outside, and a dictum is a way of commanding the outside you to line up with the inside you. It's a way of commanding your outside behavior to match up with your inside character—a way of commanding your outside achievements to rise to the potential of your inner abilities.

"But I feel as if I'm lying," Sarah said. "I just can't say, 'I *am* a thin, healthy woman today'—or any day for that matter, Coach—when I look in the mirror and can plainly see that I am a fat, unhealthy woman! Should I say, 'I *am* a thin, healthy woman *today* just waiting to emerge tomorrow'?" She spoke that last line like a drill sergeant.

She was serious so I didn't laugh, but I did smile. I asked, "Sarah, what *can* you say with all honesty about who you are on the inside? What is your character when it comes to losing some weight and feeding your physical body better nutrients?"

Sarah thought for a moment and then said, "Coach, I think I'm a disciplined, committed woman who can take control over what she eats."

"You just think you are?" I asked.

Sarah knew what to say: "I'm a disciplined, committed woman who can take control over what she eats."

"Can or does?" I asked.

Sarah responded, "I'm a disciplined, committed woman who takes control over what she eats."

"When?" I asked.

"Today!" she almost shouted.

"You really *are* that person?" I asked.

She strung her dictum all together in a highly forceful way: "I *am* a disciplined, committed woman who takes control over what she eats *today!*" She and Art were using the same volume and tone of voice!

"Is that a lie, Sarah?" I asked.

"No!" she shouted at me.

"*That's* a dictum, Sarah," I said. "Speak that to yourself. Command that person into being, and when you command that person into being, you will find yourself taking control over what you do about food."

Who we are and what we do are intricately and mysteriously linked. The more you do something, the more you adopt an identity as being a person who does certain things. The more you have a fixed description of your own identity, the more you do things associated with that identity.

The first time Joe smoked a cigarette, for example, he didn't think of himself as a smoker. A dozen or so packs later, he probably did. Over time he saw himself as a "one-pack-a-day smoker." Today he sees himself as a former smoker. If he continues to live without smoking, he one day won't even apply the word *smoker* to himself unless somebody else brings up the issue.

As a smoker, Joe smoked. The more he smoked, the more he reinforced the identity he had of himself as a smoker. When he stopped smoking, he started thinking of himself differently. The process is cyclical. It doesn't really matter where you jump in—change your behavior, change your identity. Whichever comes first, the other will follow. The strongest approach is to change your identity first, with changes of behavior following. Dictums that are associated with the "*I am*" traits of your identity are extremely powerful change agents for behavior.

The Highest and Best You

The starting place in constructing dictums is at the highest level of what you want to be. A friend of mine identified these top four things that she wanted her family members and her colleagues to know her as:

- I want to be a consistent, faithful Christian.
- I want to be a well-respected and excellent teacher.
- I want to be a healthy, physically fit person.
- I want to be a good wife, mother, and friend.

The second step is to break down each of these "be" statements into behaviors or tasks. Ask: What does it take to *be* this type of person? or

How will I know that I'm this type of person? You may want to ask: How will other people know I'm this type of person?

Here's the way my friend broke down these categories:

A consistent, faithful Christian reads her Bible every day, prays every day, goes to church regularly, is involved in some type of outreach ministry to other people, and is free to talk to people about Jesus.

A well-respected and excellent teacher never stops learning personally, including how to be a better teacher; goes into a classroom prepared to the best of her ability; maintains a disciplined classroom; encourages students; and is a good role model for behavior.

A healthy and physically fit person eats right, exercises daily, drinks lots of water, takes vitamins, and gets sufficient sleep and relaxation.

A good wife, mother, and friend communicates well, including listening well; encourages others; nourishes others in helpful ways physically and emotionally; keeps a clean and orderly home; and prays for and with her family and friends.

Hang in there! This gets a little complicated and detailed before it gets simple and streamlined.

The third step is to identify a list of things that can be done daily or weekly to foster, instill, and bolster these behaviors. In all, my friend listed the following sixteen behaviors:

1. Pray every day (including prayer for family and friends).
2. Read the Bible every day.
3. Go to church at least once a week.
4. Be part of a ministry outreach once a week.
5. Read or learn something every day.
6. Speak encouraging words to students and family members every day.
7. Eat the right foods every day.
8. Exercise—some type of aerobic, weight-training, or flexibility activity—every day.

9. Take vitamins every day.
10. Hug and kiss spouse and each child every day—at least once.
11. Spend quality time listening to family members every day.
12. Have one meal together as a family every day.
13. Do a house-related chore every day (or major housecleaning once a week).
14. Call or e-mail at least one friend every day.
15. Go to bed at a reasonable hour every day.
16. Do something that is relaxing every day. (My friend likes to knit, so her relaxing activity was to knit for at least fifteen minutes a day.)

The fourth step is to translate each of these statements into an *I am* command.

1. I AM a prayer warrior.
2. I AM a Bible reader.
3. I AM a churchgoer.
4. I AM a feeder of the homeless.
5. I AM a reader.
6. I AM an encourager.
7. I AM a nutritional eater.
8. I AM an exerciser.
9. I AM a vitamin taker.
10. I AM an affectionate wife and mother.
11. I AM a listener.
12. I AM the hostess of my family dinner table. (She did not perform all the cooking chores; they were shared with specified family members.)
13. I AM the keeper of a beautiful home.
14. I AM a communicative and loving friend. (She later adjusted this to name a different friend by name each day. In other words, she said, I AM a communicative and loving friend to Diane.)

15. I AM a sound sleeper and a fully rested person.

16. I AM a knitter.

What a list! Nobody can handle that much at one time. I encouraged her to pare down the list to those things that she wanted to *incorporate*, *add*, or *change* in her life.

It is very important that you have at least seven dictums in each area of your Totally Fit Life program.

My friend was already many of the things she had listed. For example, she already was a well-prepared teacher who encouraged and disciplined her students naturally and positively; she already took vitamins every day; she was a sound sleeper who for years had disciplined herself to get eight hours of sleep a night; she had housekeeping and home decorating down to satisfying routines; she found time to knit every morning between a quiet time (during which she read her Bible and prayed) and watching the morning news.

Given the list of sixteen items, she was able to fairly quickly zero in on the specific habits she wanted to fold into her life—in other words, the things she felt she needed to command herself to be and do every day. She ended up with this list of seven items:

1. I AM a prayer warrior who prays for the street people by name.

2. I AM a communicative and loving friend to _____.

3. I AM a reader for thirty minutes.

4. I AM a planner and consumer of nutritious meals.

5. I AM a walker.

6. I AM a superlative hostess at my dinner table.

7. I AM the keeper of a beautiful home.

The more we looked at this list together, the more we realized that these daily dictums automatically fell into categories of the Totally Fit

Life. Prayer is part of the Spiritual Fitness center of the Fitness Star. Walking is part of Physical Fitness; nutritious meal planner/consumer is part of Nutritional Fitness. Reading is a part of Mental Fitness. Being a communicating and loving friend, and providing the nurture of a beautiful home fall into the Emotional Fitness category.

Because her family's schedule was so scattered and busy, she realized that having a family meal together once a day was not something she could establish tonight or tomorrow. Rather, it was a goal toward which she could aim during the next three months, with the cooperation of her husband. We put that goal in the Directional Fitness category.

What does this woman command herself each morning? Well, we're back to the top in big-priority goals. She says in an authoritative voice:

I AM a committed Christian who prays for the street people I feed.
I AM an excellent teacher who reads for thirty minutes a day.
I AM a physically fit person who power walks daily.
I AM a healthy person who plans and eats nutritious meals.
I AM adjusting my family's priorities so we can have a meal together.
I AM a loving friend to _____.
I AM the keeper of a beautiful home.

Each of these dictums is written on a separate three-by-five-inch card. She carries these in her purse and reads them aloud as she drives to work each morning. Actually, after the first week, she had them memorized so she said them aloud as she sat at red lights in traffic.

How long did she speak these specific dictums? Until they were established habits in her life—in other words, until these habits were so firmly in place that she didn't even have to think about them. At the end of every ten-week cycle of goals, you should reevaluate your dictums. You may want to delete some, add some, and change some.

Now, how long did it take my friend to come up with these various long lists, and then pare them down? Exactly fifty-eight minutes. She considers it one of the best-spent hours of her year.

You may be asking, Why do I have to go through all of those long, detailed lists before I get to the top few dictums?

Two reasons. First, the long list will reveal how many behaviors you already have in place toward the life you want. That's rewarding and motivating. Second, the long list reveals in a personal way how behaviors are linked to character formation. That's a valuable insight.

Speak in a Command Tone

You have a "command" tone of voice even if you don't think you do. If you are a parent, you most definitely have a command tone. It is important that you speak these dictums to yourself in an out-loud command voice because what you are doing is speaking to your own soul—not to your mind. You are speaking to your emotions and your will. You are commanding yourself to *want* to be this type of person even as you are commanding yourself to do the behaviors that lead to inner character development.

Speak your dictums at least once a day, perhaps more. The frequency of repeating your daily dictums is up to you. I highly recommend that you speak your dictums in the early morning, before you get caught up in responsibilities that involve other people.

These dictums set the tone for your attitude during a day. They reinforce the character qualities you desire to have and display to others. Over time, dictums help you become the person you most want to be!

KEYS TO LASTING CHANGE

The keys described in this chapter—framing goals in a ten-week cycle, becoming part of a Team of 3®, and speaking daily dictums—are keys to developing *lasting* changes.

Liz said to me one day, "I think I'm too old to change, Coach. I'm pretty set in my ways."

Liz was a very conservative gal—she dressed in rather bland slacks and blazer outfits with her hair pulled up into a bun at the back of her neck. She didn't wear much makeup, but she was pretty enough not to need much makeup. She hardly ever smiled, but she was faithful in going to the gym to work out three mornings a week. She was intrigued with the idea of a Totally Fit Life and attended a weekend seminar about the program.

"Do you like your ways?" I asked.

"Hmmm," she said. "Most of them I *do* like."

"Is there anything you want to change for the better?"

"Yes," she admitted.

"Focus on those things," I suggested.

A few months later Liz came to see me. She plunked down a very large polka-dotted purse on my desk. It was mostly bright pink, had sequins, and the face of a poodle was on one side of it. "I've changed!" she announced.

Liz was only fifty-eight, so I didn't think I was dealing with dementia. "What are you talking about?" I asked.

"Well, you told me to focus on a couple of things I wanted to change for the better," Liz said. "I came up with five things. This purse helped me change all five things!"

"OK," I said. "How?"

"Well, I decided that since I work as a computer programmer for long hours every day, I needed more exercise in my life, more laughter, more friends, less worry, and better nutrition."

"Those are five very big goals," I said. "Good goals; Totally Fit Life goals. But what's with the purse?"

"Every afternoon at three o'clock I stand up and tell my coworkers that I'm going out for a late lunch. I grab this purse, which is a sure sign to everybody that I'm not the least bit worried about what they think of me, and I walk very quickly five city blocks to a smoothie place and order a protein shake with fresh fruit in it. I eat my nutritious mini-meal with my purse sitting on the table in front of me.

"The purse causes me to smile. I've noticed it also causes other people to smile. Sometimes people say something like, 'That's a pretty crazy purse' or, 'Where'd you find such a neat purse?' and that gets a little conversation going. I've met several people who were interesting enough to see for dinner later in the week. One of those people has started going to church with me, and I think we're going to become good friends. So—this purse has helped me exercise more, laugh more, make new friends, get better nutrition, and worry less."

Not bad for a bright pink, polka-dotted poodle purse.

"Do you think the changes are lasting?" I asked.

"Yes," she said seriously. "I probably won't carry this purse down to the smoothie place for the rest of my life, but I've learned a huge lesson with this purse."

"What's that?"

"I'm *not* completely set in my ways. I can change—and I can change for the better."

Liz plugged into a Team of 3® and began to speak daily dictums a couple of months later. She's now on her third ten-week cycle of goals with her team. I noticed recently that she had a rather large leopard-style tote bag with feathers on it. It made me smile, but mostly because I knew it made *her* smile.

COACH'S CLIPBOARD

I'm a coach, and coaches give their players specific exercises as a part of workout drills. So . . . here are your exercises for this chapter!

Commit today to a ten-week plan.

Exercise: Pick a start date. Mark off ten weeks on your calendar. (If you sign up to the Team of 3® on our Web site, this is already done for you: www.teamof3.com.)

Set your goals for the next ten weeks.

Exercise: Revisit your goals and notes from the previous chapter and begin to establish some ten-week goals for yourself in each area of the Fitness Star. Don't write in ink. You may want to revise this list as you read the next several chapters.

When three people share a common set of goals, they each are much more likely to achieve their personal goals.

Exercise: Link up with a Team of 3®.

(If you need help with this, visit our Web site: www.teamof3.com.)

A dictum is a firm commitment, rooted in a conviction, that what you are pronouncing is going to happen.

Exercise: Begin to identify "I AM" dictums related to the type of person you want to be.

Go through the exercise that is outlined in this chapter:

- Choose the descriptive words you want to mark your life. Choose three to five traits that you want as your reputation or identity.
- Identify several behaviors associated with each descriptive word or trait.

- Break down these behaviors into specifics.
- Turn these behaviors into character qualities.

Repeated behaviors become habits, and repeated habits become character.

Exercise: Begin to pursue your goals every day.

Exercise: Report your progress daily to your Team of 3® members.

Exercise: Begin to voice your "I AM" dictums every day.

TOTALLY FIT LIFE TRUTH

All things that are truly beneficial happen *over time* . . . *with* other people . . . and flow from the *inside out.*

CHAPTER 5

Rev-Up and Rebalance: Physical Fitness After 40

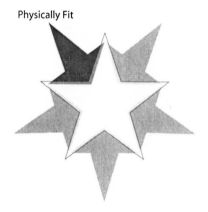

Physically Fit

I thought I'd gradually grow old gracefully," Bethene said to me. She quickly added, "No way."

"But you are a very gracious woman," I responded.

"No, I'm not," Bethene said. "I'm a bumbling, still-trying-to-find-my-way forty-seven-year-old mother of two children who are in college, and for twenty-five years I've been wife to a husband I'm still trying to figure out. I feel as if every day I'm getting slower and slower. Suddenly the clock strikes nine o'clock at night, the day is over, and I've done only half of what I had intended to do. And the sad truth, Coach, is that it is half of what I used to be able to do in a day! Most nights I collapse into bed feeling worn out, and I often wake up the next morning still feeling worn out. There's absolutely nothing 'graceful' about slowing down and wearing out."

I stood corrected.

People after the age of forty are faced with the challenge of reversing a general trend of "slowing down" and "wearing out." The reversal starts in the mind. Many people over the age of forty question whether they can rev-up and replenish. The good news is that in many ways, the declines associated with aging can be slowed, and in some cases reversed!

There's good reason to hope on many fronts. Some of the people I know in the fitness world refer to the "bounce back" factor. People who are bouncing back are people who have decided that they are going to give up former bad habits and pursue greater health. There's also the "get in gear" category. Those who fall into this group are people who were never in very good shape when they were in their twenties and thirties, who suddenly decide that they are going to get in shape in their forties, fifties, or older years. I've met countless people in the bodybuilding world who took on the challenge of bodybuilding after they turned forty. Their results are amazing.

The good news for you today is: You *can* be healthier by this time next year. You *can* be stronger, more flexible, and have greater endurance by this time next year. You *can* have more energy by this time next year. And you *can* see some appreciable and measurable objective differences in ten weeks!

Many people who decide to pursue the Totally Fit Life program begin at the point of physical fitness. Often it is a physical condition that drives people to confront their lives and decide to make changes. Some people come to the program because of a physical condition, ailment, or disease. They may be struggling with obesity, or be in recovery from surgery or a heart attack. Others are like Bethene—they simply don't have the energy they used to have.

REDEFINING PHYSICAL FITNESS IN "AFTER 40" TERMS

Most people I meet need a new definition of physical fitness. Physical fitness is not a matter of exercise, or any one particular type of exercise. Exercise is a *part* of what is required for physical fitness—it is one method of becoming more physically fit—but it is not the total sum of Physical fitness. Here's the definition I use:

> *Physical fitness is having the energy and strength you need to do all the things you want to do or believe you should do.*

The Totally Fit Life program is aimed at helping you become stronger, have more energy, and see improvement in your overall health. It is a program that can be pursued by a person at any age and sustained for the rest of the person's life. Let's look first at four words: *health, strength, flexibility*, and *energy*.

Health

To be healthy means to be free of disease and factors that contribute to disease. For many people after the age of forty, improvements in health come by reversing old "intake" patterns. By midlife, many people have developed patterns of intake that are deeply ingrained, even to the point of addiction. These patterns, however, are ones that culminate in much higher probability of degenerative, debilitating, "suffering" diseases. The time to start the reversal process is *immediately*. Very specifically:

If you are smoking, you need to stop smoking. Stop taking nicotine and the tar of smoke into your lungs and bloodstream. Plain and simple, smoking significantly increases your risk of heart disease, lung cancer, and a host of other cancers. (Some researchers estimate that smoking is correlated to 30 percent of all cancer deaths.) Smoking damages health even if a person smokes only an occasional cigarette or cigar.

Can a person stop? Yes. There are countless programs to help you. Step down and cold turkey programs both work—if you work them. Just about everybody I've ever met who was a former smoker has told me that three things helped greatly in quitting.

First, they had the support of their family and friends—support registered as encouragement, not nagging. Second, they ate a diet rich in fresh fruits and vegetables. The cleaner and more whole the food, as in fresh and raw, the less the person had a desire to smoke. And third, exercise became a priority. Aerobic exercise, especially, helped clear out the lungs and improve lung capacity over time. Initially, walking, jogging, or swimming were motivating because these air-intensive exercises revealed the extent to which they did *not* have sufficient lung power. After a while, however, these exercises were motivating because they gave an endorphin infusion that felt good—replacing the nicotine fix that had also made them feel good in the past.

The bounce-back factor for stopping is very good. A person who is smoke free for only a year reduces his or her excess risk of heart disease by half. After fifteen years of being smoke free, the risk of cardiovascular disease is similar to that of a nonsmoker's. After five years of being cigarette free, the risk for lung cancer decreases to *half* of what it was when the person smoked. After ten years, the fatality risk for lung cancer is on par with someone who never smoked.

If you are overweight, lose the excess weight. Adjust your intake of food. And make a decision that you are not going to be a yo-yo dieter—a person who gains and loses the same fifteen pounds repeatedly. Studies have shown that people who lose ten pounds—regardless of their starting weight—lower their risk of high blood pressure and diabetes. They also cut in half their risk for osteoarthritis. There's more in the chapter on nutritional fitness about weight loss, but at this point, recognize that yo-yo dieting can lower long-term immune function and excess weight can greatly increase the risk of numerous degenerative diseases. If you have an intake problem with food, identify it and reverse it.

If you drink alcohol in excess, or take any other chemical in excess—prescription or nonprescription—stop doing what you are doing. Large amounts of alcohol kill brain neurons—alcohol consumption that raises blood alcohol levels to 0.08 or higher, generally five or more drinks at one time, can be damaging. Alcohol can also cause fat to accumulate around the liver and lead to cirrhosis (or scarring) and other types of liver disease, including liver cancer.

Drug addiction, including overuse of prescription medicines, is harmful at any age, but *especially* after forty. The body's tissues are less capable of dealing with artificial chemicals—in many cases, people over the age of seventy are taking too many medications and too much of them not because of any initial error on their part, but because medicines have been added to their health-care regimen over time without a thorough appraisal and periodic reappraisal by a qualified physician, pharmacist, or pharmacologist.

Balance intake and output. Bill was forty pounds overweight when he started going regularly to a gym. He complained to me three months after he had taken out his gym membership that he hadn't lost a pound, even though he had been very faithful in exercising for forty-five minutes, five days a week. He said, "The only change I see is that I'm more tired."

As we conversed, two things became apparent. First, Bill was exercising. He was building up muscle and losing fat. Muscle weighs more than fat, so although Bill hadn't lost much on the scales, he was converting bad fat into good muscle. Second, Bill had done nothing to change his consumption pattern! He was doing well on the *output* side of exercise, but had done nothing to alter his *input* side of eating. In fact, he had somewhat convinced himself that doing all the exercise gave him license to eat just as much as he had been eating before, if not a little "extra" to help him get over feeling so tired and depleted after an exercise session.

Input and output always need to be in balance for health. This is true whether you are talking about exercise and eating, working and sleeping, giving and receiving, learning and applying, or any other form of input and output.

Not only is it important for you to address negative *intake* patterns in your life, but also to address the overall balance between intake and output.

Reevaluate your "ontake" factors. In addition to intake, you may also need to address factors related to what I call "ontake." People tend to take on more and more responsibilities, commitments, and tasks as they move through life, and by midlife the amount of ontake can be tremendous. These same people, of course, expect to be able to take on additional responsibilities and commitments and accomplish the tasks related to them in the same amount of time, which means that specific tasks are ones they expect to do in less and less time.

As a nation, we are getting less sleep than we used to get twenty years ago—per person, on average. As a nation, we are also doing more and more tasks in a given day than we were attempting to do twenty years ago—per person, on average. The result is a nation of people who have taken on too much and are drowning in stress and an overuse of antacids, pain relievers, and sleeping tablets. Our immune systems are suffering, our degenerative disease rates are climbing, and we are feeling less fit all the time.

No amount of exercise can completely de-stress a person. Exercise can help—not only in defusing stress but also in helping a person to sleep more soundly. But exercise alone cannot de-stress a person. You must address the ontake factors of your life if you are going to live in balance.

- Get enough sleep—seven hours minimum per night. Try to identify what is optimal for you. Some people need eight hours; some people need nine. Some people think they need less sleep the older they get. That isn't always the case. Some people need more sleep.
- Reevaluate your memberships, commitments, and obligations.
- Reevaluate your schedule in any given day, week, and month. In some cases, you may need to employ some serious time-management skills to dramatically revise schedules and routines. In some cases, you may need to push out your goals—trying to achieve too much in too little time can be counterproductive. In some cases, you may need to postpone some activities and goals. As a friend of mine says, "You can have it all in life—you just can't have it all at the same time."

Know what you need to know. When it comes to your health, ignorance is not bliss. You need to make certain as you grow older that you are getting periodic health checkups. There are some general health tests you need to start having at age forty—and preferably from age thirty-five:

- For women: annual Pap smear (or once every two to three years if tests are consistently normal and you are sexually monogamous), as well as annual pelvic and breast exams
- For men: a prostate exam as a baseline, and then periodically as test results warrant
- Blood pressure tests every two years, and more frequently if a physician identifies a need
- Annual dental exam, and twice-yearly teeth and gum cleaning
- Cholesterol screening every five years, and more frequently if you have elevated cholesterol levels
- Skin examination by a health-care provider every three years unless you have skin problems, have had any form of cancer, or

have the potential for problems such as those identified in the segment on sun exposure. In those cases, you may need an annual skin examination by a dermatologist.

- Baseline thyroid test, followed by repeat screening every five years
- Baseline mammogram for women, followed by one every one to two years until age fifty, and annually after that

After the age of forty-five, you need to add:

- Eye exam every two to four years
- Fasting blood sugar test to check for diabetes
- Fecal-occult blood test to check for colon and rectal cancer
- Baseline bone-mineral-density test (especially after menopause for women), and periodic bone-mineral-density tests depending upon what the baseline test shows

Strength

A second key word associated with physical fitness is *strength*. This refers not only to your ability to work, lift weights, or finish a task in the short term but also to your endurance over a longer period. Generally speaking, the stronger a person's muscles, the greater the person's ability to complete both short-term and long-term tasks.

Keep in mind as you read through the next several paragraphs that the heart is a muscle. What you do to exercise other muscles of the body is also beneficial to your entire cardiovascular system: heart, lungs, and blood vessels. If you want one muscle to be strong—with enduring strength—it's the heart muscle!

Several things are required for muscles to become strong or stronger. The muscle cells must have sufficient fuel—generally in the form of glucose provided from either fat-storage cells or food sources. Just as is true for the gasoline required by a high performance sports or luxury car, the body needs top-grade fuel to function at its best. Check your nutrition. Make sure you are getting the best fuel for health. (There's more on this in the Nutritional Fitness chapter.)

The muscle cells must have sufficient oxygen. In order for muscle cells to have sufficient fuel and oxygen, the transportation system of the body must be in good working order—in other words, there must be good flow of oxygen and fuel to the muscle cells by way of the bloodstream.

During exercise, muscle cells release toxins and take in fuel and oxygen. The toxins are carried away in the bloodstream, and it is therefore important that the kidneys and intestines and colon are also in good order so these toxins can be eliminated from the body. Some of the toxins released by physical tissues during exercise are also released through the skin in the form of perspiration.

Strong muscles are vital for overall strength of the body to do work. But a healthy digestive system, liver, cardiovascular system, and elimination system are also vital for the creation of strong muscles. Keep this in mind as you prepare to exercise. Your body is a complex and interrelated system. Lifting weights, walking around a track, or using various pieces of exercise equipment have great benefit in helping you become stronger—but these exercises are beneficial *in relation and in proportion to the health of your overall body.*

Aerobic exercises. There are two types of exercise that build up strength. Aerobic exercises are those that increase the flow of oxygen in the cardiovascular system. A friend of mine refers to these exercises as the "huff and puff" exercises—exercises such as walking, jogging, running, aerobic dancing, synchronized swimming exercises, swimming laps, cycling, and so forth. Aerobic exercises are especially beneficial for the heart and lungs. They make the heart muscle stronger.

Work with a qualified trainer or exercise-physiology expert to determine how much aerobic exercise you should do at a time. This is especially important if you are recovering from a heart attack or have been diagnosed with any type of cardiovascular or lung-related disease or condition. Most people can work their way up to thirty minutes of aerobic exercise three to four times a week. Start out at a slow pace the first five minutes, exercise at a rate that is optimal for your body mass index, and then slow the pace the last five minutes for a cool-down.

If you have joint problems with your knees, ankles, or hips, you may find that swimming is the best aerobic exercise for you. This is also a preferred form of exercise for people who are developing arthritis. Make sure you exercise in a warm pool. Also keep in mind that swimming is *not* of great benefit for people who are developing osteoporosis. You need the pull of gravity to help build up bones.

Studies have shown that doing thirty minutes of aerobic exercise in ten-minute sessions, three times a day, can be as beneficial as one thirty-minute workout, so there's very little justification for the "I don't have time" excuse. I recently heard about a grandmother—age fifty-three—who took her grandchildren to school each morning. When she dropped them off, she took a turn around the track adjacent to the school playground for fifteen minutes of walking. Later, when she went to pick up the children at the end of the school day, she took another turn around the track. The grandkids joined her for the afternoon walk. This was a good time for them to talk over the school day and also for the kids to burn off some of their pent-up energy. Good for Grandma!

In doing shorter periods of aerobic exercise, make sure you get up to a pace that puts you in your optimal heart-rate zone.

If you are obese, do your aerobics at a slightly slower pace for a slightly longer period. You'll get as much benefit—some studies show more benefit—because people who are obese tend to walk more if they are not required to walk as fast.

Weight-training/resistance exercises. Weight-training exercises are exercises that build up specific muscle groups. These are also called resistance exercises. Ideally, you will be doing each of these two types of exercises three times a week. I recommend that you alternate—do aerobic exercise one day, weight-training exercises the next day.

Work with a qualified trainer to determine exactly which weight-training exercises are right for you. Most personal routines will have a balance of upper body and lower body exercises. Also work with your trainer to determine your starting weights for each type of exercise, and the number of repetitions and sets you should be doing.

More movement. In addition to aerobic and weight-training exercises, try to build more movement into your life. If you work in a multistory office building, take the stairs instead of the elevator. If your office is at the top of a high-rise building, take the stairs at least part of the way. If you go to the mall or grocery store, park as far away from the mall entrance or store entrance as you can, not as close as you can. Walk the dog yourself, rather than relying on one of your teenagers to do it. Get out and play catch with your grandchildren rather than watching them from the patio.

Keep in mind that exercise can do a great deal to help you if you develop lower back pain. Exercises such as walking build up bone and muscle. Stretching exercises can do wonders. Many lower back problems are the result of tight hamstrings, the biggest muscles in your body, and tight piriformis muscles, which run through the gluts. Stretching these two muscle groups can greatly minimize lower back pain for many people.

Also check the way in which you lift items. Be sure to bend your knees and squat, then keep your back straight and hold the item close to your body as you lift it.

Keep in mind that you don't need to go to a gym to exercise. There are lots of items around your home—from chairs to full water bottles—that you can use in developing a weight-training program. Resistance-training exercises cause you to use your body as "weight"—for example, sitting or pressing against a wall in your home. Simple exercise equipment, from stretching bands to jump ropes, can be used at home. You can also lace on your walking shoes and walk around the neighborhood, or get back into the habit of riding a bicycle. (You may have had great fun riding your bike as a child; you can enjoy that activity again!)

You can work out to exercise videos or DVDs—these are available with workouts that range from simple to intense, some have music and dance steps, and some are at the level of drill sergeant intensity when it comes to motivation.

Flexibility

As people age, they tend to become less flexible, and in some cases, less mobile. Much of this is because as people age they tend to take on jobs and tasks that are more and more sedentary. One of the disadvantages to being promoted to a "supervisor's desk job" is the fact that a person is now sitting down eight hours a day and pushing paper, rather than doing the more physically intense work required by the frontline work!

Exercises that you once may have called "calisthenics" or "stretching exercises" can help keep you flexible. Again, work with a qualified exercise trainer or coach to develop a series of exercises that will be most beneficial for you—including the number of repetitions and sets you should do in a given workout session.

Flexibility exercises are best combined with aerobic or weight-training programs. Do your stretching *after* your muscles are warmed up a little. For example, walk for several minutes before stretching leg muscles. Stretching immediately after working out will greatly reduce lactic acid buildup the following few days.

Energy

Contrary to what many people think, exercise does not deplete energy. It adds to energy! A friend told me recently that several years ago, she was greatly annoyed when a physician advised her to develop an "exercise habit." She said, "I told him, 'Listen, Doc, I'm exhausted already. I don't need to be doing more, I need to be doing less.' He just smiled at me and said, 'Do less for your children and do more exercise for yourself.' Let me assure you, Coach, I resented that—but he was right."

This woman began to go to a gym close to her home and, because she liked to swim, she got involved in a swimming class—a combination of exercises in the shallow end of one pool followed by swimming laps in an adjacent lap pool. She said, "I found that after swimming, I had a real surge of energy that got me through the evening."

"What about doing less for the children?" I asked.

"What my physician meant was that I needed to let them help with house and yard chores. I got them busy out in the garden and assigned them housekeeping chores that actually turned out to give them some physical activity they hadn't been getting while playing videogames and watching television. Once we had fully settled into a new routine of more activity, we discovered that we were all sleeping better and feeling better."

Exercise seems to boost energy levels especially if it is done in the early morning—before the first meal of the day. Drink a little water before you head out to exercise and then consider having a protein-and-fruit shake for breakfast about thirty minutes after you quit exercising. Make a large shake and take half of it with you for a midmorning snack. (You might want to add some vitamin C granules to the shake to keep the fruit from turning brown.) You may be surprised how adopting such a simple exercise-eating routine can boost your energy level all day.

Other tips related to energy and nutrition are in the Nutritional Fitness chapter. For now, recognize that exercise *generates* more energy than it expends.

SUSTAINING A PHYSICAL FITNESS PROGRAM

People often have difficulty sustaining an exercise program. Let me address the four basic issues involved.

Variety

Put variety into your program. You may want to walk for a couple of months, then swim for a few months, and then bicycle for a few months. For years I led groups in exercise, and I don't believe any person or group ever did *exactly* the same workout twice. I always jumbled up the sequence of exercises and the number of repetitions for various movements. Occasionally we changed the normal rules of a game or added something that made a particular movement more difficult. That made the workout more fun, and when people have fun at exercising, they tend to stick with exercising! The more variety you have in a workout, the less "burn out."

Daily Exercise

Do *something* six days a week. Exercise needs to be done daily, but not every type of exercise needs to be done every day. I recommend doing three days of cardiovascular aerobics exercise and three days of weight-training (resistance-training, strength-training) exercise—alternating days. Do flexibility exercises after aerobics exercise or weight-training workouts.

Groups

Your exercise group may be your Team of 3®. It may be a group exercise class at a local pool or gym. Working out with a group of people has great benefit. Not only will you enjoy the social camaraderie—again, if the exercise is more fun, you'll exercise more—but you'll get good exercise tips from other people in the program and you'll be more motivated to continue with the program.

Get to know some of the people at the gym or in the exercise class. The more you know people, the more you'll enjoy being with them. Talk to your family members or Team of 3® partners as you walk together or do flexibility or strength-building exercises. Use your exercise time as friendship-building and family-building opportunities.

Charts and Logs

Keep track of your progress in a graphic way with an exercise log, chart, graph, or some other means that gives you a quick visual overview of what you are doing and what results you are achieving.

If you can see progress, you'll feel satisfaction and motivation simultaneously. Some of the charts may be related to your exercise program; others might deal with general health factors such as blood pressure, cholesterol levels, weight, or body-mass-index scores. The progress that is most important to me as a coach is showing up! (Charting is available to Team of 3® members on our Web site: www.teamof3.com.)

These four elements—variety, daily exercise, participation in a group, and keeping a chart or log—are essential for sustaining a program. They are the elements that make a program both fun and rewarding. It's human nature to do, and continue to do, what is fun and rewarding. Make it true of your physical fitness program!

Practical Tips

Let me give you six very practical tips:

1. *Don't compare yourself to anyone else.* There's always somebody who can lift more, run faster, or climb more steps. There's always someone who looks better in gym shorts than you do. Exercise for *you.*

2. *Wear clothing adequate for the activity.* Having good quality clothing and gear doesn't mean you need to invest a lot of money. Good shoes with sufficient support are a must for aerobic exercises such as walking, running, and dancing. If you are a swimmer, invest in some goggles to protect your eyes from the chlorine, and possibly ear plugs. If you are a cyclist or like to Rollerblade—and yes, lots of after-forty people Rollerblade and do it very well— wear a helmet and protect your knees and elbows. If you exercise outside, dress in layers that you can put on and peel off. If you

exercise before dawn or after dusk, wear reflective tape or clothes with reflective strips—or wear light-colored garments.

3. *Avoid pain.* The old adage "No pain, no gain" just isn't healthful. If you push yourself to the point of pain, you likely are injuring muscle tissue. Or if you are pushing yourself at aerobic exercise, you are likely to suffer strains or shin splints. The end result is that you won't be able to exercise that muscle for a while. That's counter-productive. If you feel pain, stop immediately.

4. *Don't eat right before you exercise—or right after exercise.* This is especially important if you desire to lose weight. If you exercise right after eating, your body will use the food for fuel instead of burning fat reserves. The most effective exercise for burning fat is done about three hours *after* a person eats, or first thing in the morning before breakfast. After you exercise, take time to cool off, shower, and get dressed. The first half hour after you finish your workout is the optimal time for the body to burn fat.

5. *Stay hydrated.* Be sure you drink adequate water before and after exercise. If necessary, carry a bottle of water with you on your walk, and definitely on your cycling trips. In fact, if you are walking, consider carrying two bottles of water—one in each hand. They act as weights!

6. *Work with a trainer.* I mentioned this previously. Too many people launch into an exercise program without adequate information. If you haven't exercised in a while, have special physical needs, are seeking to lose weight, don't want to become injured, don't know how to use certain pieces of exercise equipment, have never done stretching exercises or used weight-training machines; if you are just coming out of rehab from surgery, heart problems, or injury; if you have diabetes or heart disease; if you want help toning a particular part of your body; or if you are *more than forty years old*—work with a trainer!

To find a good trainer, ask someone who uses one or go to a reputable gym or workout center. Health facilities that are linked to a hospital usually are good in helping you with a baseline assessment of your health conditions and exercise needs.

Overcome the Inertia of Excuses

If you are over forty, you should know by now that all of the excuses people use for not exercising are bogus.

"I don't have time"—well, we do what we want to do. You can always make time. Get up a half hour earlier, turn off the television, don't talk so much on the phone, eat out less, or use your lunch break for exercise instead of eating. Every person can carve out twenty to thirty minutes in a twenty-four-hour day. If you can't, you're too busy and are likely suffering from stress.

"I get enough exercise on the job" is invalid because no job, no matter how strenuous the lifting and toting might be, exercises all parts of the body. No job provides an adequate balance of aerobics, weight-training, and flexibility exercises. Even the professional athletes with whom I've worked exercise apart from their sports-related workouts—especially during off-season times.

"I'm busy all day, so I must get enough exercise." Activity and exercise are two different things. Activity—such as taking a flight of stairs—may use up a few extra calories, but it doesn't necessarily have an aerobic effect.

"I play golf on weekends." Good, but not genuine exercise, not even if you carry your own bag, which very few people do these days. Weekend-warrior sports enthusiasts are often prone to injury because they don't regularly exercise to build muscle tissue, gain flexibility, or improve their cardiovascular health.

"I'm too old." Nobody is ever too old to start doing *something* that can help with cardiovascular health, flexibility, or muscle strength and tone.

"I'm too sick." Very few people reading this book are too sick to make significant changes that will help improve their situation, including some form of movement or exercise.

Nope—there are no acceptable excuses.

PHYSICAL FITNESS GOALS FOR A TEN-WEEK CYCLE

I strongly encourage you to do the following as you set goals for your Team of 3® for a ten-week cycle:

- *Be realistic.* Don't expect to swim a mile, walk three miles, or lift a hundred pounds your first day out. Don't aim for a world record after a month. Be realistic, but at the same time, challenge yourself. Start at a level that a colleague of mine describes as "You probably can accomplish this with some effort."
- *Seek gradual improvement.* Begin where you are and seek slow growth. Recognize that not all growth is steady. Growth tends to come in spurts, and plateaus—times when you don't progress but hold your own—are likely.
- *Establish rewards.* Don't reward yourself with food or a "day off," but do reward yourself with fun. Don't wait for the "big accomplishment" to give yourself a reward. Set rewards for incremental goals. You might reward yourself with a headset or CD player so you can play music as you walk or a new piece of gear for your bicycle. Choose rewards that motivate you toward future exercise.

PHYSICAL FITNESS AND YOUR TEAM OF 3®

Your foremost responsibility to your Team of 3® members is to set goals. I recommend minimal goals of doing six days per week of exercise, making a daily report to your team partners, and being a fountain of encouragement.

As an encourager, keep in mind that people often experience a tremendous barrier after they've been exercising for a few weeks, especially if they haven't exercised in a while and are just resuming a new physical fitness program. If you are with team partners who are newcomers or recent returnees to physical fitness, be especially encouraging!

As a Team of 3®, your accountability to one another depends on the fact that you are active—generally on a good, fair, none scale. You can define "good active" and "fair active" among yourselves in any way you like. "Good active" might be thirty or more minutes of aerobics exercise, a full set of weight-training exercises, flexibility exercises along with aerobics and weight training, or participation in an exercise class. "Fair active" might mean going to the gym for *any* form of exercise, or doing less than thirty minutes of aerobics.

I recommend that you report to your Team of 3® partners what kind of exercise you did. On our Web site (www.teamof3.com), we provide a "narrative journal" opportunity for Team of 3® members for just this purpose. If you reach a milestone accomplishment, such as, "I walked a full two miles for the first time today" or "I walked a mile in less than twelve minutes today" or "I swam eighteen laps at the pool today—my first quarter mile"—feel free to share that achievement.

If you actually meet to exercise *with* your Team of 3® partners, set both ultimate goals and incremental goals. You might want to consider establishing a group reward if you make your goal—perhaps going to a movie or concert together. (Do *not* invest in concession-stand foods while you are there!)

Feel free to share with your Team of 3® members various tips that you acquire about exercise, exercise equipment, or about overall health factors. A woman said to me not long ago: "One of my Team of 3® friends suggested that since we were walkers, we define *activity* according to the number of steps we took. I had never heard about a pedometer before, but we each bought one. 'Good active' for us was eight hundred or more steps in a day, and 'fair active' was less than eight hundred steps but more than five hundred. That sure did keep us from cheating on our self-evaluations of what was good or fair!"

"Was that motivating for you?" I asked.

"Very," she said. "I felt that I had a really good reality check at the end of each day. I found myself saying in the early morning, *I'm going to get eight hundred today!*"

Which brings us to dictums.

DICTUMS FOR PHYSICAL FITNESS

It is very important that you have dictums in the physical fitness area of your Totally Fit Life program. Command your body into motion! Below are a few possible dictums. A complete list of suggested dictums is in the Appendix. As I recommended in a previous chapter, state your personal dictum or dictums aloud and with force!

Possible Physical Fitness Dictums
1. I AM physically fit.
2. I AM an active person.
3. I AM strong.
4. I AM energetic.
5. I AM healthy.
6. I AM flexible.
7. I AM full of vitality.

COACH'S CLIPBOARD

I'm a coach, and coaches give their players specific exercises as a part of workout drills. So . . . here are your exercises for this chapter!

In what ways do you need to adjust your *intake*?

Exercise: Review the intake patterns in your life. Reflect on ways to eliminate the negative patterns and to address your overall balance between intake and output. List them here.

In what ways do you need to adjust your *ontake*?

Exercise: Look at your personal set of responsibilities, commitments, and tasks. Are there any you could or should set aside? List them here.

What medical tests do you need to schedule to have baseline "numbers" related to your physical health?

Exercise: Make an appointment!

How might you improve your exercise of these types?

Aerobic exercise:

Weight-training exercise:

Flexibility exercise:

How might you add more general activity to your life?

Exercise: Identify three to five ways to add more general activity to your life.

What are your personal fitness goals and rewards?

Exercise: Set specific and realistic fitness goals for the next ten weeks. Make a note of them here.

Have you established dictums to help set your body in motion?

Exercise: Establish dictums to support your physical fitness goals. Choose some from this book or create your own. Make note of them here, and speak them daily.

Be accountable to others.

Exercise: Report your progress in your activity level to your Team of 3®.

TOTALLY FIT LIFE TRUTH

Your body is the only body you are going to have for the rest of your life. What you do with it *today* will greatly impact the quality of life you enjoy today . . . and tomorrow.

CHAPTER 6

Refocusing Your Target:
Directional Fitness After 40

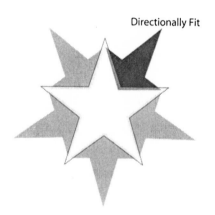

Directionally Fit

I have a lot of energy and I'm pretty fit," Harriet said. She looked fit, and she was munching a big, fresh green apple, which I took as a good sign. "I've got great friendships. I eat right. I love God. I have a great job."

"Hey, what more do you want?" I asked cheerfully. Obviously there was something more that she wanted out of life or she wouldn't have been standing in the doorway of my office.

"When people ask me what I do, I'm a little embarrassed to tell them because the next thing they say is, 'That sounds great,' and in truth, it isn't—at least not in my opinion," she said. "I'm going to be forty next month. I should be doing something that I personally think is *fantastic*."

I asked a few more questions and learned that Harriet was married, but her husband was in the military and had been on overseas assignment for most of the last two years. They agreed when they married that he'd do the moving about and she'd keep the home she had purchased. In other words, Harriet wasn't expected to pack up and move every few years from one military base to another. Her husband was in the military as a career and was getting close to the twenty-year mark. They eventually hoped to retire on some property they had purchased in Utah.

Harriet worked as the marketing director for a consulting firm that worked with major retailers across the country. She previously worked for a major communications company in marketing and steadily climbed the corporate ladder until the consulting firm offered her a job, salary, and challenge she couldn't resist. She had been employed with the consulting firm for about four years, enjoyed her work most of the time, but was unchallenged by it. When it came to developing marketing plans, conducting focus group studies, and preparing trend charts she had a pretty jaded "been there, done that" attitude.

"Let's see," I said. "You're nearly forty and you don't know what you want to do when you grow up. Have you given any thought about what you really *like* to do? What is the one thing that makes you pound the table with excitement? Apparently marketing doesn't incite passion in your heart anymore."

"Actually, I don't think it ever did," Harriet said. "I got a job in marketing right out of college, and I was good at what I did, so I got promoted and the more money I made and the better I got at what I was doing, the more I got promoted, and the more money I made and so forth. It just happened. I've been in marketing for seventeen years, I'm good at what I do, I make a good income, but I don't really *care* about marketing. Last year's products are next year's old-fashioned has-beens. It's a steady grind that doesn't produce anything lasting."

Harriet is not unlike a number of forty-something people I've met through the years who don't like their lives. They have a nagging sense that they aren't really fulfilling their life's purpose, and they have a slight but growing fear that they are going to wake up one morning and ask, *Is that all there is?* and then die in dissatisfaction.

A good job isn't necessarily a fulfilling job. A good career isn't necessarily satisfying. A good set of memberships in all the "right" clubs and organizations isn't necessarily meaningful. People crave what *counts*. They want a slice of the truly important things in life.

"I think it's all the hero movies," Mrs. Kenter said. She came to the gym that I owned when she was seventy and I was forty. I would have felt silly calling her anything other than Mrs. Kenter. She had a strong theory that people were running themselves ragged and getting overstressed because they weren't satisfied with an "ordinary" life.

"In the movies," she said, "people are always saving the world. On most days, I just try to keep my roses alive and make sure I remember to put out a little bowl of milk for the stray cat that comes to my back door."

"But you haven't lived an ordinary life," I pointed out. Mrs. Kenter was married to a wealthy man who died ten years before I met her. They had traveled the world together and met countless people in numerous ports. She had stories of experiences to last for more hours of conversation than I was ever going to be privileged to have with her.

"It was ordinary from where I sat," Mrs. Kenter said. "I got up each morning and fixed my husband breakfast—or at least I ordered it from room service. I made sure he had clean underwear and socks. I had lunch with my girlfriends when I was home and not traveling with Walt on business. I learned to pump gasoline into my car and even sack up my own groceries. You have to be satisfied in life."

"Did you ever get bored, or feel as if you were in a rut?" I asked.

"No," she said, and I knew she meant it. "I had my charity."

"What was that?"

"I was a patron of the library," Mrs. Kenter said. "I ordered books and purchased them for the local library. I helped design and outfit two mobile libraries. Sometimes I helped out at the library cataloging and shelving books. But mostly I helped organize and run literacy programs for poor children. I taught them to read—usually after school, and in some cases instead of school. We lived for many years in an agricultural area that had migrant workers helping with the crops, and some of those migrant children never did get to go to school with regularity. I taught the older ones to read, I read aloud to the younger ones, and I gave them books."

Mrs. Kenter had a cause, a passion—a reason for getting up in the morning.

"But you traveled so much," I said. "How did you manage to do all that?"

"We traveled a lot, it's true," Mrs. Kenter said. "But we were home at least half of any given year. While we were on the road, I took book catalogs with me and planned out the books I was going to buy for the library and to give away personally."

Mrs. Kenter knew that I am a Christian; she is a Christian as well. She said, "Coach Don, I know you'll understand when I tell you that one of the books I read to the children and had them read to me was the Bible. I gave away probably ten thousand children's Bibles through the years to migrant children and poor children in our area and in other places. When we traveled overseas, I always tried to locate a Bible publisher in that area so I could buy Bibles and have them delivered to poor churches. Several times I arranged for Bibles to be shipped to people who had never seen a Bible."

"That isn't ordinary," I said to Mrs. Kenter. "That's extraordinary! It wasn't saving the world, but it was making the world a better place."

"But isn't that what ordinary people should be doing?" she said.

She had a point.

I asked Harriet if she ever thought about volunteering at the local library. She was puzzled, naturally, so I proceeded to tell her about Mrs. Kenter.

"There are two big questions you need to answer that Mrs. Kenter answered for herself years ago," I said to Harriet. These are the two questions I gave her:

What makes your life meaningful and satisfying?
What do you still want to accomplish?

By the age of forty most people know a little something about what they *don't* want to do. Several years ago I decided that I was bored with what I was doing, and I decided to do something else. I went through some difficult times because I made some changes and decisions too abruptly and without enough wise counsel. But I ended up where I am today, and for that I'm grateful. What I am doing today gives my life meaning and satisfaction—and I'm never bored. Knowing what you *don't* want to do can give you some clues about what you *do* want to do.

You are likely to find that you have the most meaning and satisfaction in your life if you do the following things:

- Perform tasks and activities that are fully in keeping with your inherent, God-given-from-birth talents and traits. People find meaning in doing things they are uniquely gifted to do.
- Employ skills that you have developed to some degree of expertise. People are fulfilled in doing things they are good at doing.
- Use your talents and skills to help or uplift other people. People find meaning and fulfillment in helping other people.

- Use your talents and skills in helpful and uplifting ways alongside people you enjoy being with. People find great satisfaction in working with teams of like-minded people.

Donald is an acquaintance of mine. He is a musician—a guitarist, singer, arranger, and on occasion a composer. He's always been musical and always been involved in music in some way. Being musical is a God-given talent he's had from birth. He loves to perform but recognized early on that there aren't many professional guitar-singer opportunities apart from being a rock star or pop singer, neither of which really interested him. So, for more than thirty years, Donald has worked in a music store and taught guitar, and during the past ten years he has sung on Thursday and Saturday nights at a very nice restaurant. He enjoys his life, but the thing that really gives Donald purpose and meaning are his commitments to playing the guitar and singing at various retirement homes on Sunday afternoons.

He takes some of his students with him to entertain the "old folk"— some now younger than Donald. He enjoys the opportunity to perform with his students, and to see them perform for the residents of these retirement centers. He loves playing old favorites for the people, including old gospel songs and tunes that were popular in the 1940s.

Donald has always found satisfaction in playing the guitar and singing, even if he was alone on his back porch. He experienced satisfaction in earning money and building a good reputation and career in the local music industry. He has discovered *great* satisfaction in giving away his music, especially to people who needed to hear his music, and with people who appreciate the opportunity to perform.

I suspect that's the formula that works for just about any talent that is turned into a skill through practice, training, and education, and then is given—in cooperation with other givers—to help people in need.

What makes *your* life meaningful and satisfying? If you haven't answered that question yet, perhaps you need to take a long look at your inherent talents, skills, and the ways you might use them as part of a cooperative group helping people in need.

THE MIDLIFE CAREER CRISIS

Harriet heard and responded to what I said about Mrs. Kenter, about Harriet's talents and skills, and about the need for using her talents in a cooperative effort to help others. "The only problem, Coach," she said, "is that I don't know what my real talents are. I need to know what they are before I can develop them and use them, right?"

Right.

I am amazed that people do get to midlife without knowing what they are good at, but it happens fairly often. I asked her, "What have you always found easy to do?"

"Draw," she said.

I was surprised, but continued my line of questioning. "What do you like to draw?"

"Still lifes—you know, bowls of fruit and flowers," she said, "and buildings."

"Are you good at drawing?" I asked.

"Yes," she said. "People have always said so, from the time I was a little girl."

"Then that's it!" I said. "You were born to be an artist."

"Well, I'm not *that* good," she said.

I sent Harriet to a company in our area that specialized in aptitude tests. They were fairly expensive tests, but Harriet was thrilled at the idea of discovering her *real* talents. She came back a month or so later with great enthusiasm. "I wasn't born to be an artist, Coach. I was born to be an architect!" she said. "I've already talked this over with my husband

and he's excited about it. I imagine he thinks I'll be able to design our dream home for free. Anyway—I'm going down next week to enroll in architecture studies."

She did. And four years later, Harriet graduated with honors from a very well-respected architecture school. By that time, she knew the kinds of buildings she wanted to design. Most were portable structures that could be used in remote areas. She had designed them to be solar or wind powered, with simple water-purification systems attached to them. She saw them as useful worldwide, constructed on a modular basis for maximum flexibility. With her great sense of design and artistic flair she adapted her designs for these structures to various cultural styles.

Given the superb marketing skills she developed through the years, she's already well on her way to getting the funding she needs for full manufacturing of the buildings. She's especially excited to see how they might be used as temporary housing in times of environmental crises, such as tsunamis, floods, or hurricanes. Not only is Harriet excited about her future, but her husband is also eager to help her work with various government and military leaders in determining how these portable housing units might be used in nation-building efforts.

Harriet knows what she wants to do with her life!

If you are in a career or job today that seems dead-end, boring, or without meaning, give some thought first and foremost to the following:

- What you are good at doing
- What you like to do
- What you find natural and fairly easy to do with some degree of success
- The area of your God-given talents

And then seek out ways in which you can develop those talents!

DIRECTIONAL FITNESS

"I understand physical fitness," Larry said, "but directional fitness? What on earth is that?"

Very simple! Directional fitness comes down to this:

Directional fitness is moving intentionally and consistently toward the accomplishment of a set of goals that are meaningful.

What direction is your life taking? Do you like that direction? Are you in a career that is going toward goals that you personally find exciting and potentially fulfilling?

You are responsible for defining your own goals, because you alone know what talents you have, what skills you have or can develop, the ways in which you might use your talents and skills, and the people with whom you might employ your talents and abilities to help others. You alone know the passion that lies at the bottom of your own heart.

For most people who are over forty, the second question noted earlier in this chapter is the question that looms before them: *What do I still want to accomplish in my life?*

THE UNFINISHED TASK

Lots of people in our society are caught up in planning for retirement. It seems that's especially true for those in their fifties. Some people think in terms of their hobbies. They see retirement years as a good time for traveling, fishing, playing golf, having more time to read, and so forth. Others think in terms of the legacy they still hope to leave behind.

In my experience, fifty is the magical milestone birthday that causes many people to say: "I haven't really done anything important yet" or "I haven't done what I've always dreamed of doing."

There's greater urgency after fifty to get things accomplished or started—perhaps it's a sense that a person is running out of time to make an impact. I know very few people who hope to impact the world and leave a lasting mark in history. I know lots of people who hope to impact their families, or one sector of their community or church, and leave a legacy to the next generation.

Whether you think big or small, and no matter what type of impact you hope to make or the nature of the legacy you hope to leave, you will be dealing with issues of directional fitness. What do you wish you could do more of? What do you hope to give more of? Whom do you hope to impact more directly or with greater force? What do you have a passion for accomplishing?

It's on the issue of passion that lots of people get hung up. Even people who had a great passion for making goals in their twenties sometimes seem to lose that passion by the time they are forty or fifty.

"I wish there was something to light my fire these days," Bill said to me. "I just don't seem to have as much get-up-and-go as I once had."

I suggested to Bill that the clues to what might reignite his passion were already there. They were there primarily in his personal checkbook, his calendar, and his recurring complaints about the things in life that irritate him the most. These same clues may also help you reignite a passion.

First, take a look at your checkbook. What do you spend your money on? Especially look at your expenditures in the not-a-necessity category. What are you excited about finding on sale? What do you scour catalogs to find?

Second, take a look at your schedule. What do you schedule things around? What part of the week do you look forward to the most?

Third, consider what irritates you. What do you see as problems? Irritation with a problem or sadness over a need is very often an indication that you have a desire to see that problem eliminated or that need solved on a scale that is bigger than your own life. The greater your irritation or sorrow, the greater your desire is likely to be to take positive action aimed at solutions.

If you don't have a passion after doing those three things, root around in your life until you discover one. The point is that you need to have something in your life that you are excited about. You won't have much of an interest in sustaining the hard work of pursuing the Totally Fit Life—especially in areas of exercise and good nutrition—if you don't have something that you'd like to continue to do with energy and health for the next ten, twenty, thirty, or more years.

FOCUS COMES FROM PURPOSE AND PASSION

When you have a purpose and a passion, you'll have a focused reason for getting out of bed on Monday morning! A person with purpose plus passion is a person who is energized to do well in life and is eager to be as "whole" as possible in order to accomplish as much as possible. The people who are most successful in developing a Totally Fit Life are quick to give me reasons such as the following for pursuing the program:

- "I have a lot to do, and I need to stay fit to do it."
- "I don't want to retire—I want to recharge and continue working until I'm a hundred!"
- "I want to get over this injury and get back to what's important to me."

The formula looks like this:

$$Passion + Purpose = Focus$$

Focus, in turn, fosters motivation and momentum. People with a reason for living and a zest for living don't need to be talked into doing the right things physically, emotionally, or attitudinally for maximum well-being. They *want* to do those things. They are motivated to make the most of their lives and, therefore, to do the things that will enable them to make the most of their lives.

It's not a mystery. It's not complicated. It's not even tough to do. When you want to pursue a passion and a purpose, you will also want to stay focused on wholeness. You'll be motivated to pursue the things that help you reach your ultimate goals. When a person is focused and motivated for long enough, momentum kicks in. Goals are reached with greater speed and ease. There's something of a snowball-rolling-down-a-mountain effect.

GETTING TO THE NEXT LEVEL

When you pursue goals related to purpose and do so with passion, you have a much greater likelihood of taking your life to the next level. You need to recognize, however, that there's always a certain amount of opposition to anything that is forward-moving or upward-bound in a person's life. You will never be beyond all obstacles, detours, or delays.

Obstacles are those things that stand in the way of your progress. They must be overcome.

Detours are enticements that get you off the path of your true purpose to pursue things that seem interesting. Detours may prick your curiosity and be fun for a while, but for the most part, they are counterproductive to reaching your main goals. Avoid them.

Delays are time constraints or resource-related limitations that keep you from moving forward as quickly as you would like. Wait out delays with patience and resolve, and make good use of the time and resources you *do* have to further develop or practice purpose-related skills.

Obstacles, detours, and delays can include some of these factors:

- *Laziness.* We all have days when we'd rather relax and let life happen. A day or two of that is fine. In fact, a periodic "break" in the hot pursuit of your goals is recommended. (See the section on Ten-Week Cycles in Chapter 4.) A month or two of laziness, however, is dangerous. A year or two is disastrous.
- *Exhaustion.* We all tend to overwork or overdo at times, s ometimes to the point of great weariness. Take a break before you totally burn out—otherwise you'll find it difficult to get back on track. If you are routinely exhausted, find out why. You may need some medical help, a readjustment in your priorities and number of commitments, or practical help in overcoming stress.
- *Illness or Accident.* We all get sick or injured in little ways, and sometimes in big ways. Get well or recover as quickly as you can. Don't let an illness or accident begin to define you as an invalid or as a purposeless human being.
- *Competing Interests.* From time to time, we all find ourselves becoming interested in things—activities, groups, events—that are not directly related to our passion or purpose. We tend to dabble in hobbies and "try on" various organizations or memberships. The people who truly succeed in fulfilling what they believe to be their life's ultimate purpose are people who have an ability to come quickly back to the central focus of their life and pull all other interests toward that central core.
- *Major Life Events.* Major events—normal and to be expected— can distract a person from his purpose. Such events may be joyful or sorrowful. Babies are born, people die, children leave home, people marry, jobs and careers begin or end, children graduate, retirement comes, and so forth. These events do not need to

derail your purpose or passion, however. You may need to make adjustments, and generally you can.

- *Natural Catastrophes and Other Environmental Events.* I have no doubt that Hurricane Katrina, 9/11, or any number of other catastrophic events impacted many people's pursuit of goals! Not only do such events impact the people immediately affected, they also impact people a great distance away from the event, in financial, psychological, emotional, and spiritual ways. From time to time, we each must recognize and accept the fact that the universe doesn't run according to our wishes, will, or wristwatch. To a certain extent, we need to go with the flow—at least long enough to get our bearings and find a way to continue the pursuit of our goals.

FLEXIBILITY AND PLEASURE IN THE JOURNEY

"It sounds like a lot of work." That was the summary statement Rick made after hearing a presentation on directional fitness. "Where's the fun?"

I responded, "Having passion for doing what you do *is* fun!"

"I hear you," said Roger, "but passion sounds so *intense*. Aren't there any times in which you can just kick back, relax, and enjoy the sunset?"

Absolutely. I do not want to give you the impression that the Totally Fit Life is totally void of pleasurable moments. To the contrary! At times, just sitting and staring into space is entirely appropriate. So are spontaneous get-away weekends with your spouse, showing up unexpectedly at your junior-high granddaughter's school to take her out to lunch, and stopping to watch the neighborhood kids play baseball on the diamond at the park. Not every moment of life needs to be planned out or intentional.

Directional fitness has to do with setting big goals in life—goals of purpose that incite your own passion—and then creating and managing incremental goals so that you ultimately fulfill the reason for your life. When the "big picture" of life is in focus and the majority of your activities, resources, and commitments are aimed at the accomplishment of the big goals, the small moments take on a special quality all their own.

There's even more pleasure in sitting down to a giant scoop of praline pecan ice cream if this is the rare exception to your otherwise well-executed nutritional fitness program. There's tremendous pleasure in sleeping in after completing a major project or business trip that moved you closer to your ultimate goals. There's joy in picking up the phone and spontaneously calling a friend to talk over issues big and small, without any thought to how long the call might be. Such a call may be just what you need for emotional fitness. You don't need, however, to say about every call you make, *This is part of my emotional fitness program.* To a certain extent, take life as it comes and enjoy it! As a friend of mine said, "Enjoy the melon and spit out the seeds."

DIRECTIONAL FITNESS AND YOUR TEAM OF 3®

The extent to which you share your reason for wanting to pursue the Totally Fit Life, and the extent to which you reveal your purpose and passion in life, is up to you. The more you get to know your Team of 3® partners, the more you may desire to share what motivates you. If a team member shares purpose and passion with you, be encouraging to the extent that you can be. If the purpose and passion of that person are in any way offensive to you, or disturbing to you, you might encourage the person to rethink or reevaluate those goals.

For example, you can say, "Hey, you really seem into this. Are there other things that interest you?" or, "Do you have a plan for using this passion to help other people?" or, "I've never known anybody who was so passionate about that. How did you acquire this passion?"

Perhaps the more you know about the other person's purpose or passion, the more you will either understand the person or find a way in which you might influence him to pursue something even more positive, beneficial, or helpful. Keep in mind, too, that if you share your passion and purpose with others, you are giving them extra fuel to use in motivating you. That can be good if you don't mind being reminded periodically that you've voiced a noble purpose or expressed a strong passion. It can be irritating if you don't want to be reminded periodically that you are being lazy, or are running down a rabbit trail away from your central purpose for living. Weigh carefully how much you want to say and to whom.

You will benefit greatly if you are linked up in your Team of 3® with people who have a degree of passion and a similar commitment to a purpose-filled goal. People who have a great passion for similar activities or causes are likely to be more encouraging and more motivating to one another than people who have dissimilar passions or dissimilar degrees of passion. People of different passions can work together on common goals, but they are less likely to become friends or stay teamed together after an initial ten-week cycle.

Marilyn, Jody, and Alexis were three forty-something-year-old women in the same Team of 3®. They found each other at a Totally Fit Life seminar weekend and realized that they had some common interests. They met together later for tea and, as they talked, they bemoaned the fact that all of the goodies presented to them at their chosen teatime café were loaded with sugar and fat. "It wasn't diet food," said Marilyn, "and we all shared a desire to lose at least ten pounds and get in better shape both physically and nutritionally."

They began to talk as they walked together about doing a tea that offered nutritional and tasty items. When Oprah and other television personalities began to speak in favor of green tea as a good beverage for nutritional and weight-loss purposes, these women decided to sponsor their first "terrific tea for total fitness" event. They got a restaurant that served breakfast and lunch to let them lease the facility for several hours one afternoon.

Each of the women went to classes to get a food-handler's license, and they worked together to make recipes in the restaurant kitchen that were very low in sugar and fat, but very high in flavor and texture. They put up flyers at a number of gyms and talked to a sympathetic reporter at a local paper. The event was a huge success. They presented information about the protocol that women love when it comes to an English tea, the history of tea, and several other topics. They made more than a $300 profit, which they donated to another thing they had in common—the need for exercise equipment at their children's private Christian school.

This tea was not a one-time-only event. They later sponsored "terrific teas" that covered Japanese tea ceremony protocol and the teas of India. The profits from those two teas were given to their children's private Christian school for mission trips by the high school upperclassmen to Japan and India. The profits from the last tea were used to buy items for the school library. Later a "terrific tea for Christmas" yielded money to buy books as presents for needy children.

These women shared a mutual passion and purpose beyond walking together! Eventually they sponsored a tea every month. And when did they do most of their planning related to these teas? On a nearby park's walking path, where they met and walked three mornings a week.

DIRECTIONAL FITNESS AND TEN-WEEK CYCLES

Directional fitness is all about *big* goals. A ten-week cycle is about tackling a chunk of that big goal. Keep your intermediate goals doable in ten weeks and set appropriate rewards for accomplishing your subgoals.

In a way, directional fitness goals impact all other areas of fitness in positive ways. If your directional fitness goals are focused, you'll have a greater motivation for setting nutritional and physical fitness goals, which aim at giving you the vitality and vibrancy you need to accomplish your major life purpose.

If your directional fitness goals are focused, you'll have a stronger desire to be emotionally and mentally in shape to accomplish those goals. Mental fitness goals have a much greater likelihood of being focused toward equipping a person with the intellectual skills and most helpful attitudes toward accomplishing big-picture goals. When it comes to emotional fitness, working toward a life-purpose goal can produce a tremendous amount of joy and hope. Personally, I don't believe it's possible to have strong *hope* if you don't have an ultimate sense of where you are going, with a reasonable expectation of arrival at the desired destination.

DICTUMS FOR DIRECTIONAL FITNESS

Directional fitness dictums go straight to the heart of your priority goals. These dictums remind you *why* you are speaking all of the other dictums! Below are some suggestions. Reflect upon who you are and what you really have a passion for doing. Reflect upon the purpose for which you believe you have been put on this earth. Be bold in writing out and speaking your dictums.

Possible Directional Fitness Dictums
1. I AM achieving.
2. I AM pursuing my life goals.
3. I AM successful.
4. I AM making a difference.
5. I AM gifted.
6. I AM building a legacy.
7. I AM passionate about my God-given purpose.

COACH'S CLIPBOARD

I'm a coach, and coaches give their players specific exercises as a part of workout drills. So ... here are your exercises for this chapter!

Are you a "natural talent"?

Exercise: Think about your natural talents. Choose at least three and write them down. (Example: A good speaking voice is a natural talent.)

Are you skilled?

Exercise: Write down the ways in which you have turned your natural talents into skills. (Example: Using your good voice as a public speaker is a skill.)

Do you have spiritual gifts?

Exercise: Identify your major spiritual gift.

(Example: you love to teach Sunday school, and you're good at it.)

Are you giving?

Exercise: Identify two or three ways you can use your talents—natural and spiritual—to benefit a group or person in need. Then pick a group to which you will give your talents.

Do you have life goals and a plan to accomplish them?

Exercise: Make a short list of your life goals. List things you see as having great purpose and for which you have great passion.

Exercise: Break this list down into ten-week goals; see how they fit inside the segments of the Fitness Star.

Exercise: Write dictums that address your life goals. Begin to voice them daily.

Be accountable to others.

Exercise: Report your progress in the area of directional fitness to your Team of 3®.

TOTALLY FIT LIFE TRUTH

What I chose to do today will take me one step closer to, or move me one step further away from, my life purpose.

CHAPTER 7

Right Eating for Repair and Refurbishment: Nutritional Fitness After 40

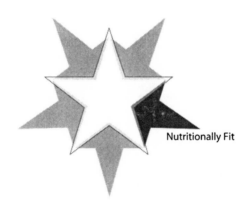

Nutritionally Fit

Ⅰf I am what I eat," Carolyn said to me, "then I'm half Italian food and half chocolate pie." She quickly added, "Very high-quality Italian food and very good chocolate pie."

Carolyn didn't have any self-esteem problems. She was just overweight, not unlike half of the women who are forty and older. Even though we seem to be a nation that is crazed with health foods and model-perfect bodies, we are also a nation that consumes far more calories than it expends, and many of the calories we consume do nothing to promote health.

By the time a person crosses a magical milestone birthday, that person very likely has deeply ingrained eating habits. Some foods have taken on mythical identities—they have become the "I must have" and "only this says comfort to me" foods that we crave. Other people find in midlife that certain foods are now indigestible. They have developed problems that keep them from milk products, grains, legumes, lettuce, and other foods—perhaps from a malfunctioning of their digestive systems, perhaps from a slow-developing allergy to the very food they once craved to excess. The specific nutritional needs of those after forty tend to fall into three very broad categories:

- Immunity
- Energy (physical and mental)
- Obesity

Each of these issues, however, must be addressed in addition to a sound foundation of good nutritional habits. Let's begin there.

A FOUNDATION OF GOOD NUTRITIONAL HABITS

Becoming intentional about the Totally Fit Life includes becoming intentional about what you eat. I'm always amazed that when I ask people "Why do you eat?" few people have a quick answer. They eat because they eat. They have to. Their bodies need fuel. The greater answer is that we eat because we need to grow new cells or repair and refurbish the cells we have. These physical processes in our bodies continue in midlife. We still need new cells, and we need to repair and refurbish old ones. An adult who doesn't eat withers, atrophies, and shrivels. An adult who doesn't eat the right things isn't healthy.

There are also psychological factors that are related to eating—especially in our choice of foods, our aversions to some types of foods, obesity, and a "failure to eat." Although we tend to think of anorexia and bulimia as conditions that impact mostly young women, a growing number of forty-something women are suffering from these eating disorders. In most cases, these conditions are also linked to poor self-image and in more than half of the cases, psychologists tell us that these conditions are linked to previous abuse in the woman's life. If you truly want to have a Totally Fit Life, you need to honestly face the question, Why do you eat?

Back to the Basics of Our Need for Cell Generation and Regeneration

What we eat determines both the quantity and quality of the cells we create, repair, or renew. You can never be physically healthier than the quality of food and beverage that you take into your system. If you boast, "I don't have any diseases, and I've been eating junk food for decades," you need to add "yet" to your boast. Years of eating high-sugar foods, wrong fats, and too much food *do* impact health in later years. Nutritional factors account for a very high percentage of the causes of degenerative diseases, which include cancer, heart disease, stroke, and type 2 diabetes.

The basic formula for good eating is very simple:

Right Amounts + Right Foods + Right Frequency = Right-On Health!

Let's break that down.

Right amounts. Small is right; big is wrong. You intuitively know what a small portion of something is. Small is the muffin your mother made, not the one you buy today at the designer coffee shop. Some of today's muffins are equal to three or four of the size Mom made! Small is the size of the palm of your hand, not the platter-sized portion that is served at many restaurants. Small is a true eight-ounce cup, not a mug, which may hold sixteen or more ounces. The right amount for health is "small." Your body wasn't created for an excessive volume of food to be crammed through the plumbing of your digestive track.

Right foods. This is the sticky point for most people. Health producing is right; unhealthful is wrong. And yes, you know what these foods are, too. I often hand out a sheet with the information below to those attending Totally Fit Life seminars.

WHICH IS RIGHT?

Circle the food choice that you know is the "right" way to eat:

Half-pound cheeseburger cooked in grease, with a large-size order of french fries and a milkshake	*or*	Salad with tuna chunks and fresh tomatoes and lots of green veggies (such as cucumbers, snow peas, green beans, broccoli bits, and so forth) with a dressing of olive oil and balsamic vinegar
A double mocha topped with sprinkles and whipped cream	*or*	A tall glass of peach tea sweetened with Splenda
Chicken-fried steak with mashed potatoes, both smothered with gravy, and corn on the cob covered with butter	*or*	Grilled, blackened fish with rice pilaf and steamed vegetables, with fresh herbs
A piece of apple pie	*or*	A fresh, ripe apple

Nobody has ever flunked this quiz! But very few people claim to like the right way to eat. Why? Because most people have eaten high-sugar, wrong-fat foods for so long that they are addicted to sugar and fats, although they rarely want to admit this addiction. If you have eaten the wrong foods for decades, it will take time to readjust your taste buds so you will truly enjoy eating the right foods. How much time? Well—ten weeks is likely!

If you have eaten the wrong quantities of food for decades, it will take time for your stomach to "shrink" so that you feel satisfied with less food. How much time? Hmmm—about ten weeks.

If you have developed a gorge-and-snack eating pattern, it will take time for you to readjust your personal schedule to eat six small meals a day. How much time will it take to develop this new habit? I'd say about ten weeks.

You should have no difficulty setting your first ten-week-cycle goals in the area of nutritional fitness! The time to start is now. Begin to move in the right direction. Eat the right amounts, of the right foods, in the right frequency.

Right frequency. Often is right; infrequent is wrong. You also know intuitively what *often* means. How do I know that you know? Because we are a nation of snackers. We crave food multiple times a day, and that need has given rise to a huge industry of foods that are mostly unhealthful.

Many people follow this pattern: no breakfast (or if breakfast, a sugar-and-caffeine-based one), then a big lunch, an even bigger dinner, and snacks between breakfast and lunch, lunch and dinner, and dinner and bedtime. That's five to six "fuelings" a day. The wiser approach is to think six small meals a day, evenly spaced. Eat the first mini-meal a half hour after your morning exercise and continue every two and a half to three hours until a half hour before you go to bed. And eat *good* foods each time.

A balance of carbs, protein, and fiber. Each of your mini-meals needs to have some protein, a fiber-rich food, and some complex carbohydrates.

Most mini-meals also need just a little bit of fat. What you don't need in any given meal is sugar and bad fats. Let me give you a sample of some small meals that include these three foods:

- Three egg whites whipped into an omelet with nonfat cheese, half a grapefruit, and a half slice of whole-grain toast
- Three ounces of skinless chicken breast and one cup of "good" vegetables (steamed or raw)
- An apple and a half-cup of nonfat cottage cheese
- One cup of tomato dill soup with a slide of whole-grain rye bread topped with albacore tuna and a teaspoon of low-fat mayonnaise
- Two cups of Chinese vegetables stir-fried with three ounces of chicken
- A three-ounce turkey burger on one-half of a whole-wheat bun with slices of tomato, lettuce, and onion
- Two cups of mixed salad greens topped with two sliced hard-boiled eggs, and a half cup of vegetable broth
- A half cup of nonfat yogurt and a cup of cut-up fresh fruit
- Two cups of steamed broccoli, red peppers, onion, mushrooms, and zucchini topped with two ounces of plain nonfat yogurt
- A half cup of all-natural sugar-free applesauce and two links of turkey sausage (no nitrites, well-drained)
- A cup of homemade vegetable soup and a piece of cornbread (not cornmeal cake made with sugar)
- Three ounces of fish and a cup of steamed vegetables
- Half of an avocado with two ounces of albacore tuna
- Half of a pear and a half cup of nonfat cottage cheese
- Four ounces of turkey breast and a cup of steamed green beans

Incremental change. Brandon turned forty and showed up on my doorstep the next day. "I've got to do something about *this*," he said pointing to his enlarged belly. "I know there's a six-pack in there somewhere, but I don't think I've ever seen it, not even when I was a teenager." He was referring to abdominal muscles, not beverages.

I went over the basics of a good nutritional program with Brandon. He gave a big sigh and said: "I really get hung up, Coach, on the idea that I've got to change the way I eat forever—that I can never have a bowl of ice cream or a piece of pizza ever again."

I had good news for Brandon. That's *not* what is required in the Totally Fit Life program. Here's the ten-week commitment I ask people to make:

- Eat *good* four days a week.
- Eat *fair* two days of the week.
- Eat *poor* no more than one day a week.

If you can eat good four days a week, you'll be eating good almost 60 percent of the time, which is the majority of time. Over time, you will lose some weight at a fairly even pace, especially if you are exercising along the way.

When I explained this to Brandon, he said, "Okay. I suppose you are going to tell me that I already know what's good, fair, and bad."

"Of course!" I said. And in truth, Brandon knew, and so does every other person who has ever signed on to this program.

You *know* if you have eaten the right foods in the right amounts at the right frequency on any given day. You also know if you've blown it. (And if you don't have a clear vision for what that means, think "the works" pizza, a gooey dessert, a big plate of pasta with cheese sauce, or a bucket of fried chicken.)

You also know if you've had a so-so day. Fair days are ones in which you know you *could* have made better food choices, eaten smaller portions, or spaced your feedings more evenly, but you also don't feel as if you grossly overindulged.

There are four more basic principles:

- Don't have two poor days in a row. In other words, don't end one week with a bad day and start the next week with a poor day and call it a fun weekend.
- Don't store up poor days thinking that you'll have several during a week of vacation.
- Don't try to avoid all poor days. If you do, you'll feel deprived.
- Do, over time, raise your standards about what a "fair" day includes. Over time, many people find that as they lose weight and eat smarter, their formerly fair days would now be classified as poor.

Good meals begin with good foods. In order for you to eat six "good" meals a day, you need to have good food as part of each meal. Shop smart. What you don't take home, you won't find in your cupboard, and what you don't find in your cupboard, you aren't likely to eat. When you go to a grocery, shop the perimeter of the store—that's where you will find fruits, vegetables, dairy products, fish, poultry, and so forth. Stay out of the cereal, cookie, chip, candy, baked goods, bread, and ice cream aisles, and stay away from the bakery section.

Choose a wide variety of fresh foods. Try different spices and herbs. Plan your meals and always shop from a list. Be sure to keep healthful foods in your refrigerator or cupboard for snacks—such as dry-roasted macadamia nuts or almonds, olives, pepperoncini peppers, a bowl of cut-up fresh fruit, and so forth. The stronger the flavor of a "good" snack, the more satisfying it will be to you. Choose poultry and fish over red meat. Choose fresh foods over canned or frozen foods. Avoid foods with preservatives and artificial ingredients. (If you can't readily pronounce all of the ingredients on the food label, be suspicious.)

Cook smart. Eat foods fresh and whole whenever possible. If you must cook vegetables, don't overcook them. Steam them rather than boil them.

If you are cooking meat, grill it rather than fry it in oil. Don't bread or deep-fry anything! Become a salad expert, trying various combinations of fresh greens, veggies, fruits, and herbs. Make your own vinegar and olive oil dressing. Get creative. For example, make "taco" wraps using grilled chicken, nonfat cheese, and lots of tomatoes and peppers wrapped up in lettuce leaves instead of tortillas.

Eat smart. Eat slowly. Put small portions on a small plate. Allow your brain to catch up with your eating. It takes about twenty minutes for the signal to reach your brain that you've had enough.

Make smart choices at restaurants. Divide a healthful meal with another person, or immediately put half of a meal in a take-home box. Ask for salad dressing and any sauces to be served on the side. Stick to the green items on the salad bar. Stay away from appetizers and desserts—most of them are loaded with excess fat or sugar. Ask for a double portion of vegetables instead of a starch. If you order a sandwich, ask that the chef leave off the bread and give you extra tomatoes and lettuce instead. Eat only one piece of bread and butter, if any. Avoid chips and salsa if possible, or limit yourself to just a few chips and break them into tiny pieces and dip each "chipette" into the salsa sparingly.

When traveling by air, take your own food onboard.

Only go out for Italian or Mexican food once a month rather than twice a week.

Have pizza no more than once a month. Bear in mind that Italian, Mexican, and pizza consumption likely are associated with a "bad" day of eating.

Make smart choices at parties. Eat before you go to a party. Carry a glass of sugar-free iced tea in your left hand and gesture a lot. Don't carry around a plate. Choose veggies and fruit bits. If the temptation gets too great, slip away. If all else fails, plan ahead that this is going to be a bad food day and try not to make it overly bad!

Drink Plenty of Water

Most people don't drink enough water in any given day. It is very important that you keep yourself hydrated, especially when you are exercising. Keep a bottle of water nearby at all times—fill it up a couple of times a day and drink to the last drop. Most people need to be drinking eight to twelve glasses of water a day.

For every cup of caffeinated beverage you drink, drink an extra cup of water. The water in caffeinated beverages doesn't count as part of a daily total.

Alcoholic beverages also don't count in calculating how much water you should drink. Most alcoholic beverages are loaded with calories. Even though there are some in the health care and fitness industry who recommend a glass of wine a day as part of a healthful diet, I don't recommend alcohol. Alcohol has a bad effect on every major system of the human body, not to mention the consequences in the social realm, including marriage problems, drunk-driving accidents, and rude behavior that often warrants an apology. The benefits of wine lie totally in the antioxidants associated with the grapes, not the alcohol. You can get the same results from other antioxidants, even a grape or wine extract that can be taken as a supplement.

THREE SIMPLE PRINCIPLES TO MEMORIZE

I recommend that people who embark on the Totally Fit Life program memorize these three one-sentence principles:

- Eat fat, get fat. Eat lean, become lean.
- Eat too much, weigh too much. Eat less, weigh less.
- Eat good, feel good. Eat bad, feel bad.

Can you reprogram yourself to eat good foods at the right frequency and in the right amounts? Absolutely.

KEY NUTRITIONAL AREAS FOR MIDLIFE

There are two nutritional areas in which those who are in midlife and beyond need to pay extra attention. They need to do their best to keep their immune systems healthy, and they need to make sure they are getting the nutrients necessary to keep their brain health high, and thus, avoid as many strokes and dementia conditions as possible.

Boosting Your Immune System

Overall good health is directly linked to high immune system functioning. Nutritionally, there is a great deal that can be done to "eat right" for good immunity.

Why is immunity so important, and especially as we age? First, it seems that older people are often more susceptible to viruses and bacteria. This is not to say that age and lower immunity *must* be linked. It means that historically speaking, older people have lower immune systems, primarily as the result of many decades of unhealthful habits. If you want to have good immunity as an older person, you need to start *now* to develop the nutritional habits that will contribute to good immunity.

A breakdown in the immune system has also been linked to a number of degenerative diseases, including conditions that cause plaque to erupt in arteries and produce blood clots that, in turn, produce deadly heart attacks and strokes. Poor immune function is nearly always linked in some way to proliferation of cancer cells. Plus, those who live in retirement communities, nursing homes, or other close living conditions come into greater contact with viruses and bacteria. Now is the time to build immunity.

In addition to eating right, you need to make sure that you have eliminated as many toxins as possible from your personal environment. Toxins weaken the immune system. Especially avoid contact with pesticides and polluted air and water. Other major enemies of the immune system are stress, smoking, excess alcohol and caffeine, drugs (including many prescription medicines), and food additives. Here are seven of the top immunity enemies:

- Sugar
- Stress
- Smoking
- Excess intake of alcohol
- Lack of exercise
- Lack of sleep
- Lack of necessary vitamins and minerals

Some aspects of the immune system, which includes the lymphatic system, bloodstream, and the digestive system, rely on specific nutrients to keep them working efficiently. For example, interferon, an antiviral and anticancer chemical that is secreted by tissues throughout the body, needs vitamin C for its production. An antibacterial enzyme, lysozyme, which is found in bodily fluids such as tears and blood, requires vitamin A for its production.

An imbalance in the immune system can cause allergies and food intolerances, which result in a release of histamine and other chemicals to drive out what the body perceives to be an invader. A variety of negative symptoms can result if too much of these substances is released. At times the imbalance can result in autoimmunity, which occurs when the body goes into overdrive and starts producing antibodies that attack the body's tissues. Diseases such as lupus and rheumatoid arthritis are examples of autoimmune diseases.

To keep the body's immune organs and cells healthy and in balance, you must eat the right foods. In addition, exercise encourages the flow of lymph fluid (which contains immune cells), and stimulates circulation (which improves the oxygen supply to the body's organs).

Below is a short list of immunity-boosting agents:

- Foods rich in vitamins A, B complex, C, and E
- Foods high in minerals, especially zinc, selenium, and calcium
- Omega-3 and omega-6 fatty acids, which are found in nuts, seeds, and oily fish
- Protein, found in lean meat, fish, and poultry
- Fiber, found in grains, fruit, and vegetables
- Maintaining a positive outlook on life
- Regular exercise
- Adequate sleep
- Sufficient "fun" in life (including plenty of opportunities to laugh and be with friends)
- Daylight (sunlight without direct exposure)
- Prayer and various relaxation techniques that counteract stress

Since this is a chapter on nutritional fitness, the following is a list of foods linked to increased immunity in various medical research studies:

Apples	Beets
Apricots*	Black-eyed peas
Artichokes	Blueberries
Asparagus	Broccoli*
Avocados	Brussels sprouts*
Bananas	Bulgur wheat
Beans (garbanzo, green, kidney, lima)	Cabbage
	Cantaloupe*

Carrots*

Cashews

Cauliflower*

Cherries

Chicken

Chicory (or endive)

Chili peppers

Corn

Cranberries

Duck

Garlic

Ginger

Grapefruit*

Grapes

Green beans

Guava

Kale*

Kiwifruit*

Lemon

Lentils

Limes

Mackerel

Mango*

Nuts (almonds, Brazil nuts, hazelnuts, pistachios, walnuts)

Oats

Onions

Oranges*

Oysters

Papaya*

Passion fruit

Peppers (green or red bell, and hot)*

Potatoes

Pumpkin (and pumpkin seeds)*

Quinoa (grain)

Raspberries

Rhubarb

Rice

Safflower oil

Salmon

Sesame seed oil

Shrimp

Snow peas

Soy beans

Spinach

Strawberries

Sunflower seeds (and sunflower seed oil)*

Sweet potatoes and yams*

Tomatoes*

Tuna (fresh, albacore)

Turkey

Watercress

Wheat germ*

Yogurt

*These foods have been shown in medical research studies to improve brain-tissue health.

Cumin (black cumin)	Mustard seed
Cayenne pepper	Nettle
Chamomile	Peppermint
Echinacea	Rosehips
Elderflower	Rosemary
Evening primrose oil	Sage
Green tea	Thyme
Horseradish	Turmeric

These spices and herbs have been shown in research studies to enhance immunity:

There are plenty of good meals that can be made using these ingredients. Be creative!

Eating for Energy and Brain Power

As people enter midlife, they tend to become increasingly concerned about retaining memory and "mind power." Certainly exercise can help keep brain tissue healthy because exercise increases the flow of important oxygen to brain cells. Many of the substances that boost immunity are also helpful in boosting energy and keeping brain tissues as healthy as possible. The prime foods for "brainpower" are antioxidants and essential fatty acids.

Especially eat foods rich in vitamins C, E, and beta-carotene. In addition to whole foods marked with an asterisk (*) in the previous list, you might also consider a couple of items that you'll find at a health-food store: cereal grass and chlorella. These are "green foods" that many people find more enjoyable if mixed with a glass of orange juice. In addition, spinach (cooked or raw), yellow squash, and olive oil have helpful brainpower ingredients.

Fats clog up the brain, just as they clog up heart-related blood vessels. Cut out all trans fats from your diet, all saturated fats from meat and dairy products, partially hydrogenated fats (present in just about everything packaged or processed), and margarine products. Choose instead oils that are fresh, unrefined, organic, and mono-unsaturated. In other words, think olive oil! Never eat or use rancid oils. Give up fried foods. When you are cooking, don't fry. Use organic fresh-ground peanut butter.

Foods high in trans fatty acids include:

French fries
Puffed cheese snacks
Deep-fried chicken nuggets and
    fish burgers or strips
Margarine
Salad dressings (other than olive
    oil and vinegar)
Tortilla chips and potato chips
Deep-fried mushrooms and other
    deep-fried vegetables and

"cheese bits," often listed as
    appetizers in restaurants
Cake
Candy
Shortening
Doughnuts
Peanut butter (most major
    brands)
Mayonnaise
Cookies

I realize these may sound like the basics of the American diet, but they are also the reason we continue to see an increase in heart disease, strokes, and brain-related diseases.

While you don't need trans fats in your diet, you do need essential fatty acids—the omega-3 and omega-6 substances. The brain is actually made up mostly of fat, but the substances needed by the brain to produce the types of fats it *needs* are alpha-linolenic acid, linoleic acid, EPA, gamma-linolenic (GLA), arachidonic acid, DHA, PGE1, PGE2, and PGE3. Don't panic. The simpler approach is to tell you where you can find good sources for these essential fatty acids in your diet: flaxseed oil, walnut oil, certain fish meats and fish oils (which can be taken conveniently in capsule form), primrose oil, borage oil, black currant oil, animal meats, eggs, and milk.

Again, a number of these can be found in supplement form—especially the oils. If you don't believe you are getting sufficient omega-3 and omega-6 fatty acids, talk to a knowledgeable person at a reputable health-food store.

Choline and lecithin are two substances necessary for good electrical impulses in the brain. You can find choline in fish and defatted soybean flour. Lecithin is found in seed oils, liver, egg yolks, peanuts, peas, beans, Brewer's yeast, cheese, cabbage, cauliflower, and green leafy vegetables.

Three substances that function as brain poisons are *aspartame* (found in many diet products and especially in those products sweetened with NutraSweet), *food additives and preservatives* (especially sulfites, nitrates, nitrites, and for some people, MSG), and *alcohol.* I realize that millions of people drink diet drinks and use alcohol. Popularity doesn't mean these are good for either body or brain, especially your brain. Learn to live without these three brain poisons.

In addition to eating the right things for good brain function, there are other things you can do to stay "sharp" as you move through midlife toward older age. These things are presented in the chapter on Mental Fitness.

WHAT ABOUT SUPPLEMENTS?

I've mentioned various supplements in this chapter, so let me say an additional word about supplements. I personally take supplements, but I don't require people who are on the Totally Fit Life program to take them. Taking pills or liquids is just one more thing to do, and most people are already overwhelmed at the challenges of eating right, exercising, thinking right, and doing all of the other "right" things in the program.

For me, taking supplements has become a normal and habitual part of my life. I know that our food sources are often lacking in many of the nutrients they once had because our soil has become depleted. Dietary surveys have shown repeatedly that between 30 and 50 percent of the total calorie intake of the typical American is made up of highly processed, adulterated, and nutrient-deficient food. There's no way to get adequate vitamin and minerals without some effort—both eating the right things, and in some cases, adding supplements.

Here are the basics I take daily:

- *Vitamin C*—a minimum of 3,000 mg. a day. To find the optimal level of vitamin C for you, start with 1,000 mg. and then add 500 mg. a week until you experience a mild laxative effect. That's the signal you're taking more than your body needs, so back off 500 mg. and consider that your "set point" for this vitamin.
- *Vitamin E*—400 IU. There's no more healthful vitamin for your heart or brain. Make sure you take d-tocopherol vitamin E, which is made from vegetable sources. (Vitamin E made with dl-tocopherol is made from petroleum by-products. Take the "l" out of your vitamin E!)
- *Vitamin B*—taken in a homocysteine-balanced complex of the B vitamins. This is the most important vitamin you can take for general brain health. You need all of the B vitamins in proper balance.
- *Omega-3 and omega-6 oils*—taken in capsule supplements or liquid supplements (including fish-oil capsules, flax oil, evening primrose oil, borage oil, and black currant seed oil).
- *Calcium*—balanced with magnesium.
- *Selenium.* In nations where the soil is rich in selenium, cancer rates are extremely low.

Be cautious in taking herbal supplements. Make sure they are from a reputable source. If you are attempting to lose fat, you may want to take supplements of chromium picolinate and lecithin.

Do not take megadoses of any supplement for a prolonged period of time without consulting a trained professional. You want an adequate amount of nutrients, not overkill.

CONFRONTING OBESITY

And now for the topic that nearly everybody over forty knows he needs to face, but doesn't want to. Dieting is no fun at any age. Perhaps the most important first step that a person over forty can take is to have a test that determines his percentage of body fat (usually skin-fold caliper testing or underwater-displacement testing). Then, take necessary action to bring that percentage into the range of good health.

Most obese people I encounter are obsessed with their weight on the scale. They are looking for a quick fix to lose weight. What many of them don't realize is that weight can fluctuate wildly on a daily basis depending on how much water a person drinks and expels. What really matters is how much of your weight is fat. Losing fat is more difficult than simply losing pounds, but it is the type of loss that reaps the most important benefits. Don't think in terms of weight loss—think in terms of *fat* loss.

I'm not going to give you a diet to follow in this book. The plain and simple truth is that if you are eating the right foods, in the right amounts, at the right times at least four days a week at a *good* level and two days a week at a *fair* level, you *will* lose fat, especially if you are also exercising regularly. How much you lose and how quickly will be determined by how "good" you eat and how much you exercise.

"You mean I don't need to count calories?" Lex asked me.

"No," I said. "And you don't need to count carbs, fat grams, or buy a scale for portion control by ounces."

"Wow," she said in awe. "This will really work? Just eat good four days a week and exercise six days a week?"

"Yes," I said, "making sure that as part of your 'good' eating plan you are eating good foods, in good amounts, with good frequency."

Lex came back two weeks later and said, "It's harder than I thought."

"I never said it would be fast or that you wouldn't struggle a little," I replied. "You are changing habits, and they are sometimes tough to change. Hang in there." Then I shared three adjustments in her attitude that I thought might help:

1. You *do* have enough self-discipline. Don't fall into the old mind game of telling yourself that you just don't have the willpower. You do.

2. You *can* accomplish a long-term goal of significant size—including a significant amount of long-term weight loss. You just need to break down your big goal into smaller subgoals. Be realistic in your goal setting, taking into consideration your age, height, and bone structure. Along with your goals, establish some fun rewards that are *not* food focused. (In other words, don't consider an extra-large supreme pizza as your reward for losing ten pounds.)

When it came to rewards, Warren said: "I can't think of anything that isn't food!" He had rewarded himself with food for so many decades he literally could not imagine anything being fun or special that didn't have calories! I suggested buying a new swimsuit, an afternoon off to drive up into the foothills and throw Frisbees with his dog, an afternoon at the ballpark watching his favorite college or semi-pro team, a minicruise of three or four days, a new computer accessory, a new CD, tickets to a concert, and so forth.

He smiled and said, "Got it!" Warren didn't choose anything I suggested. He chose new grill utensils as the reward for when he reached his first goal, and a new outdoor grill for when he reached his ultimate goal!

His goal caused me to list a whole new set of potential rewards as part of the Totally Fit Life program: a new blender for making protein shakes, a salad spinner, a juicer, a wok, a steamer, a better set of knives, new china, new glassware, new silverware—the list is endless. Tools for the proper preparation of food are not the same as rewards of food itself.

3. You *can* learn to like a more healthful eating plan. It won't happen in just a few days or weeks. It will take a while for your body to get rid of toxins, your taste buds to readjust, and your mind to get over cravings. You didn't get fat overnight, and you won't get "unfat" overnight either. Begin to think in terms of progress. Even slow fat loss is better than no fat loss at all!

The good news is that the longer you stick with a fat-loss program—combining good eating habits and exercise—the more energy you will have! You'll be amazed. Over time, and after you have achieved your optimum fat-percentage level, you will also discover that your body has taken on a new shape—more muscle and less flab. The increase in muscle is to your benefit since muscle burns more calories in maintaining itself than soft tissue or fatty tissue. You may actually begin to eat slightly bigger portions down the line because your newly developed muscles will be burning up more calories.

How long does it take for these fat-loss basics to kick in? Oh—about ten weeks.

Lex, by the way, stuck with her fat-loss program, and after thirty weeks (three ten-week cycles), she had lost the forty pounds she wanted to lose. She discovered muscles she never knew were there. She looked great and felt great.

She admitted to me, "A lot of what needed to happen was a change in the way I thought about myself and the way I thought about weight loss. I found myself adjusting goals and dictums in my emotional fitness category and mental fitness category, even more than in my nutritional fitness and physical fitness categories."

"What were some of the things you needed to change in your thinking and feeling?" I asked. She graciously wrote out a list of items and agreed to let me share this list with other Totally Fit Life program participants. I suspect these are attitude and thought adjustments that many obese people need to make:

- I needed to stop seeing myself as a failure just because I had been unable to take charge of my weight for so many years. I needed to get past decades of yo-yo dieting and convince myself, *This time I can do it.*

- I needed to learn how to handle the temptations that were presented to me almost daily by friends and coworkers who offered me delicious-looking food items. I especially needed to learn how not to offend my overweight friends who chided me for not joining in on their trips to the ice cream store.

- I needed to be very intentional about deciding in advance what I was going to order at any restaurant I entered. That way, I didn't need to look at the menu. If I started reading a menu, I was in deep trouble.

- When I found myself thinking about food, or what I was going to have as my next meal, I literally needed to say, "Stop it, Lex" and then begin to think about something else.

- I needed to start believing some things that I had stopped believing, such as, *I don't need to be overweight just because I'm over forty, I don't need to be the victim of a slow metabolism,* and *I don't need to think I'll be more prone to sickness if I don't eat everything on my plate* (something my mother said to me when I was a child).

What you think about food is very closely tied to what you eat and how much of it, which in turn is very closely tied to how fat you are.

NUTRITIONAL FITNESS AND TEN-WEEK CYCLES

The goals you need to set for yourself should be fairly clear at this point:

Establish the goal of eating the right foods. Make meal plans and then make shopping lists according to your meal plans.

Establish the goal of eating the right amounts. Eliminate as many visual food cues as you can from your life. The less you look at television commercials, billboards, and print ads that include larger-than-life, better-than-it-actually-tastes photographs of food, the easier it will be to eat smaller amounts of good foods. Develop some of your own strategies. One person I know has a habit of setting down her fork or spoon between each bite. Another person eats for five minutes and then waits five minutes before adding more food to his meal. Yet another person serves himself a mini-meal on a bread-and-butter plate or saucer. It feels like a full plate of food to him!

Establish the goal of eating six small meals a day. Talk over your new strategy of eating six small meals a day with your spouse and family members. Encourage them to join you in this.

Establish the goal of drinking plenty of water.

Establish goals related to including foods or supplements that are specifically aimed at greater immunity and brainpower.

Establish goals related to fat loss and the achievement of a lean body.

NUTRITIONAL FITNESS AND YOUR TEAM OF 3®

You will be reporting to your team members each day whether you ate *good, fair,* or *poor.* Be honest. I encourage you not to talk too much about food with your Team of 3®. The more you talk about food, the more you think about food, and generally that means the more you start *wanting* food. On the other hand, if you come up with great tips for eating good foods, eating at the right intervals, ahd eating the right amounts—or if you discover some great tips for fat loss—share them.

Those who need to lose fat especially need encouragement from their team members.

SPEAKING DICTUMS FOR NUTRITIONAL FITNESS

Speak to yourself about your new eating habits and goals. See yourself as a lean, healthy, energetic person who eats lean, healthy, energy-producing foods. Once again, make your own set of dictums. Speak them to yourself aloud and with an "enforcer's" tone of voice.

Possible Nutritional Fitness Dictums

1. I AM eating properly.
2. I AM creating a healthy body.
3. I AM drinking enough water.
4. I AM eating right-sized portions.
5. I AM eating fresh food.
6. I AM happy.
7. I AM satisfied.

COACH'S CLIPBOARD

I'm a coach, and coaches give their players specific exercises as a part of workout drills. So . . . here are your exercises for this chapter!

Plan to succeed.

Exercise: Make meal plans for a week—that's six meals a day for seven days —forty-two meals total. Make a shopping list for just the food required to prepare those meals.

Get started.

Exercise: Write out nutritional fitness dictums and begin to speak them to yourself daily.

If you're obese . . .

Exercise: Make an appointment with a qualified clinician or care provider for a test to determine the percentage of fat in your body.

Be accountable to others.

Exercise: Report your nutritional intake to your Team of 3® daily.

TOTALLY FIT LIFE TRUTH

You really *are* what you eat.

CHAPTER 8

An Infusion of Love, Joy, and Peace: Emotional Fitness After 40

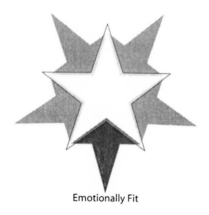

Emotionally Fit

I sometimes encounter the extremes in my work with the Totally Fit Life program. Emotional extremes are common. Some people are highly emotional. They react to life emotionally far more than they respond to life rationally. Other people run scared of their own emotions. They don't want to feel anything, much less express anything they might feel.

As in all areas of fitness, emotional fitness calls for emotions to be in balance. Emotions have been built into every person. Emotions compel us to take action, even more than our ideas or opinions compel us to act. We face the challenge of learning to acknowledge our emotions, control them, and use them in right ways. We are never, of course, to be ruled by our emotions. So what's the link to the Totally Fit Life?

People who have healthy, balanced emotions love life. They have a strong desire to be fit so they can enjoy a high quality of life for as long as possible, and they want others around them to do the same. People with healthy, balanced emotions make great friends and coworkers. Certainly every married person or parent wants his family members to have healthy, balanced emotions.

THREE GREAT OBSTACLES TO EMOTIONAL FITNESS

From my years of experience in coaching people toward a Totally Fit Life, I've learned that there are three great obstacles to emotional fitness. Nearly every person struggles at least a little with one of these obstacles at some point in his or her life. Often these struggles come to something of a climax when a person hits midlife.

Obstacle #1: Striving for Physical Beauty

I'm not opposed to physical beauty. I'm a great fan of it! But I'm also realistic about outward beauty. Physical, outer beauty diminishes with age. Any person who tries totally to deny or counteract that fact through multiple reconstructive surgeries is still going to find him- or herself or herself with an older, less physically attractive body. Gravity works—it pulls skin into sags and bags and wrinkles. Hair falls out, or begins to grow in unwanted places. Body shapes change. Chemical and hormonal changes occur.

Certainly a person can do a great deal to maintain physical muscle mass, and we can keep a body lean through a combination of nutritional fitness and exercises. A person can stay strong. I'm not at all opposed to cosmetic surgery if a person wants to pursue that. But plain and simple, there's not an eating plan, exercise program, or any supplements that can make an eighty-year-old *look* twenty.

Some people seem to hit a brick wall emotionally when they hit midlife and realize they aren't going to be as beautiful as they once were. Others have a difficult time emotionally because they are striving to hang on to something they feel they are losing in spite of their best efforts. My approach is to be as healthy as possible. Health produces a glow that *is* beautiful.

Generally, the person who strives continually for outer beauty is someone who is unhappy on the inside, with low self-esteem and deep insecurities. The effort to stay beautiful is, in part, an effort to portray a confidence and strength he or she does not feel emotionally. The person believes that if he or she *looks* beautiful, others will think he or she *is* valuable. Value has become tied to appearance, and if appearance declines, so does the person's value.

Emotional Fitness also means embracing the good news about inner beauty: it lasts! Not only does inner beauty endure, but it also has the potential for increasing as a person ages. From the Creator's standpoint, every person is beautiful, regardless of the shape of eyes, size of nose, or color of skin. Tall, short, large boned, petite—these things don't matter to God. What matters to God is that a person is the best possible steward of his or her body, rejoices in his or her uniqueness, and seeks to stay healthy, strong, and vibrant all the days of his or her life.

Obstacle #2: Striving for Perfection

Beauty is just one area of life in which people often strive for perfection. A man accused me of promoting perfectionism in the Totally Fit Life program. "Isn't your program all about a person being 'perfect'—of getting fit in every area of life in order to achieve perfection?" he asked.

No. The Totally Fit Life is about *wholeness*, not perfection. The two concepts are very different. Perfectionism is generally rooted in a *lack* of emotional fitness—it is never a hallmark of emotional fitness. The perfectionist sees what is missing *externally* and focuses all efforts upon fixing that flaw. The Totally Fit Life calls a person to look at life as a *whole* and to build wholeness from the inside out, beginning with the spiritual aspects of fitness and applying principles of identifying talents, improving skills, setting priorities, seeking balance, building relationships, and giving. Perfectionists focus on self. They rarely are great givers. The Totally Fit Life calls for a person to seek ways to build relationships and give to others.

Perhaps most importantly, perfectionism is always related to a fixed perception of what *should* be. The Totally Fit Life program is related to an ongoing growth and development toward the wholeness that *might* be. The Totally Fit Life challenges a person to drop his or her "should" criterion and to replace it with a "could" mind-set—to pursue what might be possible, what can be done, and what is worthy of pursuit.

Often when a perfectionist is faced with his or her personal failure to accomplish a specific goal, he or she abandons all goals. It's something of a boomerang effect. I've worked with people who failed to accomplish a diet goal, so they abandoned all fitness goals. I've known others who can't do the number of reps at the weights they thought they should be lifting at the end of ten weeks, who simply stop coming to the gym. These people can't cope with imperfection. If they can't do something "perfectly," they don't try to do it at all. They turn to something else they think they can accomplish to perfection.

The truth is, nobody is perfect, and we all live in an imperfect world. Nobody can achieve perfection this side of heaven. We all will die with some unresolved weakness, frailty, or flaw. That doesn't mean we should give up on life and fail to do what we *can* to move closer to the Totally Fit Life.

If you recognize yourself as a perfectionist, ask yourself the following questions:

Why do I feel a deep drive toward perfectionism?
What is it I am really trying to attain?
Who am I really trying to impress? Whose love am I really trying to win?
Why do I feel it is so important to be perfect? Who taught me that I had to be perfect in order to be loved or valued?

The emotional issues at the core of perfectionism are love, acceptance, and value. The perfectionist ultimately is trying to win acceptance or be perceived as valuable or lovable. These are the issues that need to be addressed for emotional fitness.

Jeanne came to the Totally Fit Life program after a divorce. She was forty-four. Her world had been shattered after her husband left her for a twenty-eight-year-old woman with a great body and not much evidence of intellect. Jeanne felt as if all of her life was crumbling around her, and she was clinging to anything and everything—including anyone and everyone—in an effort to control what was left of her life. She wanted to be part of the Totally Fit Life program in order to regain perfection that she felt she had lost.

She said to me with more than a little anger in her life: "If I can't actually achieve perfection, what's the point?"

I didn't mince words. "I think the point for you, Jeanne," I said, "is that you can get *well* if you pursue this program."

"But I'm not sick," she said.

"You've been injured," I countered, "badly injured. Your emotions have taken a real hit. You've been emotionally devastated by what happened to you."

Jeanne began to cry. "So what do I do?"

"First, you identify your strengths—not just your talents, but your emotional strengths. I don't know all of your strengths, but I know two of them. You are a loving mother and friend. One of your strengths is a great capacity to give love. And you are persistent. When you take on a goal, you pursue it with your whole heart and don't give up. Those are great strengths. I want you to make a list of things you are good at and traits that are emotional strengths."

She agreed. The next time we met I took a look at the list of things Jeanne had written down, and I said: "Now, develop some skills related to these things."

"How do I develop a skill related to 'be persistent'?" she asked.

"Put down next to that trait a couple of areas where you will show up and do what you set as an emotional goal, no matter how you feel or what others might say," I said. "For example, you might make a decision that you are going to show up for every one of your daughter's Little League games this summer, even if your former husband shows up."

She gulped. "OK. What about showing love? How do I turn that into a skill?"

I asked, "What is it that you do for your son and daughter that they interpret as love?"

She said, "Well, my son probably sees me as loving when I bake him chocolate chip cookies. My daughter thinks that I'm loving when I take her shopping. Both of the kids probably think of me as loving when I don't hassle them to be perfect."

I was glad Jeanne brought up that last part. She had not only been striving to regain perfection in her own life, but she had been putting great stress on her children to be perfect.

"So," I said, "bake cookies, go shopping, and cut your kids some slack. That doesn't mean you need to abandon all discipline and let them do what they want, but choose your battles wisely. They are teenagers. So what if the room isn't totally spotless or uncluttered at all times? Establish a couple of days a month when all three of you will work to clean the house and get things in order. So what if your daughter wears a little too much eye makeup at age sixteen? Consider taking your daughter to a makeup specialist so she can get her makeup information from a pro. So what if your son likes to wear torn jeans? Just insist he put them into the wash so they are *clean* torn jeans."

"OK," she said. "Then what?"

"Work on your talents; develop some new skills. Most of all, start giving yourself away, and not just to your kids. Find something to do for somebody who is in worse shape physically, emotionally, or financially than you are. And better still, do this 'giving project' with another person or a group of people. Get involved in doing something to improve the world. But remember, you aren't going to make other people or the world perfect—just better."

I had one more piece of coaching advice to give to Jeanne: "Talk to your children about the emotional challenges each of you is facing in the aftermath of this divorce. Your children are hurting as much as you are. They are facing emotional difficulties that are similar to yours, but also different. Talk it over as a family. Become something of a Team of 3® in addressing and healing your emotional wounds."

Jeanne not only got involved in a community improvement project, but she got her children involved in it as well. This became something special for mom, son, and daughter to do together. They set some goals for themselves when it came to giving. They also made a pledge to one another that they would do three things for one another: say something encouraging to one another every day, do something special for one another to say "I love you" every week, and go someplace special together—just the three of them—once a month.

The first two parts of the pledge kept love and encouragement flowing in their family of three. The latter part of the pledge helped them build some new "just us" memories on which they could reflect with joy.

About a year after the divorce, I asked Jeanne how she was doing.

She replied, "Good, Coach. Things aren't perfect—but nothing ever is, right? Things are certainly *better*, and not only that, but I have a sense they are getting better all the time."

Jeanne was on her way to *wholeness*—not perfection. She was in the process of being healed and becoming "totally fit." So are her children.

Obstacle #3: A Hunger for Acceptance and Love

Many people seem to think that low self-esteem and a deep desire to be accepted, respected, or valued by other people are issues that only the young face. Not so! These are issues that people face at all ages, and the needs and issues can be monumental in size by midlife if a person has never felt worthy, accepted, respected, or valued.

Show me a woman who is forty and has lived fifteen years in a marriage in which she feels unloved and unvalued, and I'll show you a woman desperate for love and value. Show me a man who is fifty and has never felt that his wife respected him, and I'll show you a man with a deep ache in his heart to be respected. Show me a person whose elderly parent still doesn't accept, love, or value him or her, and I'll show you a person who has emotional despair. Show me a person whose employer of thirty years cuts him or her loose with no sign of appreciation for the years of hard work and loyalty, and I'll show you a person with emotional pain.

The hunger for acceptance has sometimes been called a "love hunger." I use the word *acceptance* because I've met people who have great love from family members and friends who still have a hunger to be accepted by a particular group of people at their place of employment, in their church, or in their community. They may even like themselves, but they still have a need for someone else to appreciate their unique traits and to value their presence. Even if you call this need a love hunger, the emphasis here is on *hunger*. There's a drive, a need, a feeling of something missing, an awareness of a void that needs to be filled that is just as real as the physical sensation of hunger.

The hunger for acceptance cries out, "Love me! Value me! Accept me! Consider me worthy! Respect me! Give me dignity!" The feelings associated with this hunger are often displayed as anger, frustration, rejection, stress, discouragement, loneliness, bitterness, sadness, and depression.

Every person needs to come to a degree of healthy self-acceptance— a point where he or she sees his or her value on this earth as being rooted more in what God says than in what another person says or does. We also need to develop relationships in which someone we admire or respect says back to us: "I admire and respect *you*." We need to hear that we are loved, valued, worthy of inclusion, and important to *someone*.

The challenge is threefold. First, we must recognize that we all have this hunger for acceptance. We must own up to the fact that we cannot be emotionally isolated from the world. We need friends and people to mentor and to whom we can give. At the same time, we must take on the challenge of being a person who freely *gives* words of affirmation, respect, admiration, and appreciation to others. We must be people who are quick to say "Thank you," "I like you," "I value what you did," "I admire your stand on that," and "I appreciate your willingness to help." This level of giving and receiving—at the level of *acceptance*—is critical to your role in a Team of 3®.

The second challenge is the challenge of "appropriateness." We must give and receive the appreciation, value, love, and respect we need in ways that are healthful and helpful to others, and in ways that do not cross the boundaries of morality or propriety.

In your search for love and acceptance, don't violate your marriage vows of faithfulness. In your search for admiration and words of affirmation, don't become a cloying, clinging vine to another person. In your search for respect, don't manipulate other people to give you the compliments or recognition you think you deserve.

The end results of these behaviors can be devastating emotionally not only to you but to others around you. Seek to give and receive love and appreciation in ways that are wholesome, mutually beneficial and desirable, and that recognize boundaries of personal space.

The third challenge is the challenge of accepting the fact that no one person can ever meet all of your emotional needs, and that you will never be totally acceptable to everybody. No matter how hard you try, you will not win the affection or admiration of every person on the planet. You cannot be best friends with the whole world. You will not have the respect of every person you respect. And you cannot solve the inner needs of another person—even someone you love deeply—with outer methods, activities, and gifts. You must give emotionally to many people, and be open to receiving emotionally from many people.

Overcoming the Obstacles

The three obstacles I've identified are sometimes huge in a person's life. It is important to address any of these issues that are present in your life. Emotional fitness is directly related to the ways in which you perceive yourself as a valuable, lovable human being with a purpose on this earth.

An entire book could be written on any one of these obstacles to emotional fitness. A person may need serious counseling or benefit from intense prayer therapy or some other form of spiritual intervention. An entire family may have fallen into the traps of striving for physical beauty, striving for perfection, or becoming ravenously hungry for acceptance. I certainly don't want to downplay the importance of these needs by offering anything that might be perceived as a "quick fix." Nevertheless, given that disclaimer, I have found five pieces of advice to be very helpful to people I've met through the Totally Fit Life program:

1. *Refuse to compare.* In setting goals for yourself, don't compete with other people or compare any aspect of your life to others. If you are going to compete with anyone, compete with yourself. Set goals for yourself and work to attain them. If you find you

are comparing yourself to another person, say aloud: "Isn't that interesting? That's who they are. This is who I am." Then, point out good aspects of yourself in a noncompetitive manner.

The truth is, there's always going to be somebody who has more, achieves more, or does more. There's going to be someone who is more beautiful, stronger, more flexible, more successful, or who earns more money. Accept the reality of that! At the same time, you are always capable of doing more, having more, achieving more, and giving more. Value who you are, what you have, and what you have to give.

2. *Set realistic goals.* Perfection isn't realistic. Perfection is unattainable. Set goals that are attainable, that challenge you, and that are aimed in the direction of wholeness.

3. *Applaud others.* Don't envy the accomplishments of other people—don't covet what they have won, earned, or achieved. Applaud their win, admire their success, and appreciate their achievement. Envy can rob you of joy. Applauding others increases your own joy and makes you a person others like to be around. You'll likely find that the more you applaud others, the more others value your presence and seek to find ways to applaud and encourage you.

4. *Embrace your own uniqueness.* Discover as much about yourself as you can until you come to the firm conclusion: *I'm a Designer original.* Your Creator only made one of you, and He built into you a unique set of wonderful qualities, dreams, talents, and abilities. Your body is one of a kind. Your challenges and opportunities in any given group, at any given time, are one of a kind.

Nobody but *you* can do what you can do, when and where you have opportunity to do it, with the people God places in your path, and in the way that is distinctively your style. Embrace your distinctiveness and value the unique qualities that make up other people. In so doing, you will be valuing yourself and others. The more you value others and let them know that you do, the more you will be valued by others in return.

5. *Make friends.* Never think that you have enough friends. Never take a friendship for granted. Never think you can stop working at a friendship. There are few things in life as rewarding and nurturing as a good friendship.

THE MARKS OF A GOOD FRIENDSHIP

The people with whom you are linked as a Team of 3® have great potential to become friends, especially if you stick together for several or ongoing ten-week cycles. Keep in mind the following characteristics of real, lasting friendship.

THE EMOTIONAL BASIC 3

Through the years, I've found repeatedly that when people are asked to choose words that describe emotional fitness, they tend to choose these three: *love, joy,* and *peace.* I regard these as the Emotional Basic 3.

Love, joy, and peace don't just "happen." Nor are they fleeting. These emotional basics are rooted in intentional thought, word, and deed. These emotions take root in a person's life, and grow and flourish, when a person makes an intentional choice to do some things and to refuse to do other things.

Experiencing More Love

Love is a *verb.* It is expressed by mutual and interdependent giving and receiving. To show love, something must be given from the heart; and to feel love, something must be received fully by an open and trusting heart. Expressions of time, effort, loving words, and tangible gifts can all be perceived as love.

In saying that love is interdependent, does this mean that you can't or shouldn't show love to someone who doesn't express love back to you? No. We are called to be loving in our attitudes and actions toward all people. When it comes to real emotional bonding and fitness, however, we will find our greatest emotional strength in relationships that are *mutually* loving. In a truly loving relationship, there's reciprocity in giving and receiving. The more that is given and received, the more the love grows and develops. The more love in a person's life, the greater the emotional fitness.

What must we *refuse* in order to experience more love? We must refuse to be selfish. We must refuse to manipulate situations or people for our own gratification. We must refuse to say "mine" about all of our time or all of our possessions. We must refuse to draw attention to ourselves or seek to have all of our needs met at the expense of others who also have needs and deserve attention. We must refuse to want our way more than we want God's way.

What must we *choose* in order to experience more love? We must choose to give as many times and in as many ways as we are able to give, and as the recipient is capable of receiving. We must become good at giving five things:

1. *A listening ear.* We must choose to listen with the heart as well as the mind.
2. *Our presence.* We must choose to "show up" when another person has a loss, is ill, or experiences a setback.
3. *Applause.* We must choose to openly express our joy and enthusiasm when another person achieves, wins, or experiences a moment of success. Part of applauding other people is thanking them for what they have done for us—directly or by their examples. Choose to say thank you.

4. *Affirmation.* We must choose to build up other people by acknowledging and appreciating not only what they do but also the character traits they are displaying. We must choose to do this not only to their faces but also behind their backs, and to do so without any thought of what we might gain in return.

5. *Assistance.* We must choose to help when help is needed.

Experiencing More Joy

As stated previously, joy is not the same as happiness. Happiness is temporary; it is rooted in external circumstances and the actions of others. Happiness is highly situational and personal. Joy, in contrast, is an inner quality that is deeply rooted in a belief that life has purpose, meaning, direction, and hope.

Joy is closely linked to faith and optimism, but it is not blind faith or blind optimism. Joy is found in believing that "God is in control, and I belong to God." It is linked to beliefs that life is an awesome adventure to be enjoyed, creation is magnificent and delightful, music is to be sung, feet are made for dancing, and friends are among God's best gifts.

What must you *refuse* in order to have more joy? Refuse to give in to the impulses of despair, discouragement, and depression. These emotions will all come and will come in varying degrees. You must choose to say no to all chemicals that might alter your state of mind or cause you to have artificial highs and lows. You must refuse to develop addictions to habits and substances that do not produce a healthy body, mind, or relationships.

What must you *choose* in order to have more joy? Choose to give thanks to God for His many blessings. Choose to express appreciation and thanks to others for their gifts and kindness. Choose to praise God not only for who He is to you personally but also who He is permanently and forever—to all people throughout all ages. Choose to smile and whistle. Choose to sing songs that you make up to express your delight in living. Choose to write poems about things or people you like, admire, and value. Even if you never share your songs or poems with others, they can be a reminder to you that there is much reason for choosing to give thanks and praise on any given day.

Experiencing More Peace

Peace is not synonymous with the word *quiet*. Peace is not simply getting along with other people. It is not the mere absence of war. Peace is an inner state of tranquility and contentment that is the opposite of striving, arguing, contending, or wrangling. It is the opposite of anger, and perhaps more importantly, it is the opposite of stress-based fear.

Through the years, I've encountered dozens of people who have told me they were stressed out. Stress is the product of anxiety—of trying to do too much in too little time with too few resources. Stress has physical, mental, spiritual, and emotional dimensions. In the emotional area, stress is directly related to worry and anxiety, which are "garden varieties" of fear.

Some people are anxious or worried because they fear they won't accomplish what they are expected to accomplish in a given time frame. They are fearful they won't measure up or survive. Some people are fearful that they will never marry or will never marry again; won't measure up to the standards set by a boss, coach, or teacher; or won't survive in today's market. Saying yes to peace is very often the result of saying no to fears such as these.

What must you *refuse* in order to experience more peace? You must say no to people who insist that you do more than you can do, spend more than you have to spend, or schedule more than you have hours in a day. And that includes messages that say you must use a certain product, drive a certain type of car, or wear a certain type of clothing. Refuse any categorization or label associated with status and acceptance that is contrary to what God says about you as His beloved, valued child.

What must you *choose* in order to experience more peace? Choose to have faith that God is in control of all external circumstances and situations at all times. Choose to have faith that there are things you can do to better manage your own schedule. Choose to develop your talents and skills and then to give them away. Choose to create a peaceful environment for yourself and others. How? Here are some practical suggestions:

- Turn down the volume. Don't only reduce the noise level inside and outside your home, but turn down the volume of your own voice.
- Dim the lights and see the world by a little candlelight occasionally.
- Slow down the pace. Take some time to sit and stare, to reflect, to contemplate, to dream, to think.
- Get away from the crowd and spend time with just one person or a few friends, or by yourself.
- Turn off the electronic devices and spend time with people.
- Invite others to join you for relaxing times—talking, playing simple games, sharing experiences.

Because you can choose your emotions, you also have the ability to change your emotional response and to develop new emotional habits. You don't need to respond to an insult with anger, you don't need to respond to rejection with an insult, and you don't need to respond to negativity with sarcasm or criticism. Emotional habits develop because we fail to take charge of our habits—to recognize the good habits and grow in their expression, and to recognize bad habits and choose to change them.

Choosing is at the heart of setting emotional fitness goals, selecting and speaking dictums, and doing activities that promote love, joy, and peace in your life.

TOP 1™ MIND-SET AND ACTIVITIES

Love, joy, and peace, because they are ultimately choices that compel active behaviors, all find expression in a simple strategy that I call

"TOP 1™." This is an acronym that means: The Other Person FIRST.

TOP 1™ does not mean that you seek to "top" another person in a competitive way. TOP 1™ does not mean putting yourself as number one. It means just the opposite. TOP 1™ means that you make another person number one—by doing a simple act of loving-kindness with joy and with an intent of producing peace. TOP 1™ is

Putting another person first by showing *love* to that person by giving something to the person with *joy* and with an intent of promoting or producing *peace*.

TOP 1™ means doing something *intentional* to express kindness or love. It is the doing of a specific, identifiable, concrete act that blesses another person. It is a deliberate and conscious act of the will. It may be a word spoken with kindness, a gesture—such as opening a door, making a phone call just to say thank you, or letting a driver move into your lane without honking your horn; or a deed—such as the giving of a gift or showing up to help on moving day.

TOP 1™ is a simple act of kindness expressed with joy—with a smile, a word of praise, a note of optimism in your voice.

TOP 1™ acts are intended to make the world a little better place on any given day. They are aimed at lowering stress, alleviating fear, inspiring confidence, resolving problems, and generating a sense of well-being.

I highly recommend that you make a list of people to whom you intentionally choose to show some act of kindness every day. Include the following people in your list:

- Your spouse
- Each of your children
- Your parents if they are still living—or perhaps a sibling

- Your boss, secretary, or a specific partner or colleague
- Specific friends

In naming these people as TOP 1™ recipients, you will be much more likely to make sure you do something to show love to each of these people every day.

"Just one act of loving-kindness a day?" another person asked.

Certainly not—at *least* one act of loving-kindness a day. One loving act a day, done with joy and for the purpose of peace, is not the limit. It's the starting point! I encourage you to increase the number, magnitude, and quality of your TOP 1™ deeds. Seek to become increasingly generous, thankful, loving, joyful, and giving. I also encourage you to increase the variety of people for whom you do one TOP 1™ deed a day.

Perhaps the greatest TOP 1™ acts are those that you choose to do for people who have an adversarial relationship with you, or the person you find difficult, annoying, or problematic. The person may not regard you as an enemy, and may not even know he is at odds with you. That's the very person who can benefit most from a TOP 1™ act, and in the process of your doing TOP 1™ acts, you will likely find that your attitude changes and your frustration level declines.

The person you choose for a TOP 1™ word or deed may be someone who is very different from you. It may be a street person you see every day at the entrance to your condo complex, or a janitor who comes nightly to empty the trash in your office.

I strongly encourage you to find a child to whom you might express TOP 1™ words and deeds, even if you personally do not have a child or no longer have your children close to home. There's something especially wonderful about modeling love—with joy and with the intent of peace—for the next generation.

I also encourage you to find an older person to whom you might express TOP 1™ words and deeds, even if you don't have living parents, grandparents, or aunts and uncles. There's something very rewarding about honoring and respecting your elders.

If someone notes your TOP 1™ action and says "thank you" or "how nice," encourage that person to pass the good word or good deed forward.

Above all, don't express TOP 1™ words or deeds with an expectation that others will like you more or do something nice for you. Give generously. That's true love. Give joyfully and cheerfully. Give with peace as your motive.

TEN-WEEK CYCLES FOR EMOTIONAL FITNESS

When it comes to emotional fitness, the basic element of goal ssetting in the Totally Fit Life is to do one TOP 1™ activity every day. Keep the emphasis on practical and generous. Keep the attitude joyful and the purpose one of promoting peace. Do one TOP 1™ activity for every person on your list.

Every ten weeks evaluate your TOP 1™ list:

- Should another name or names be added to your list?
- Are there ways in which you can do more to put the other person first?
- Has a particular phrase or deed become commonplace to the point that you have less meaning for it? You may need to find creative ways to say: "I love you," "I appreciate you," or "thank you." In what ways might you be more generous, more spontaneous, more expansive, or more direct in your expressions of loving-kindness?

There are some instances in which Team of 3® members have determined among themselves that they are going to express TOP 1™ words and deeds to the same list of people. This has been very effective in corporate and church settings in which all of the team members are part of the same company or church. I recently heard about one Team of 3® who took on their "grumpy boss" as their TOP 1™ project. This guy never knew what hit him! The nicer and more helpful these joyful, peace-loving women were to him, the nicer and more helpful he became—and he never even knew it.

Not only did the entire department benefit, which included nearly thirty people under this man's supervision, but his family also benefited. His good behavior at work became his good behavior at home. The loving-kindness he received, he passed on to his wife and children, and they, in turn, impacted others. He became a role model to his children of a no-longer-grumpy, appreciative, loving, joyful dad.

EMOTIONAL FITNESS AND YOUR TEAM OF 3®

The level of accountability about TOP 1™ words and actions is very simple: yes or no. Either you've done a TOP 1™ activity in a day or you haven't.

You certainly should feel free to share creative ways in which you have expressed love. Give your Team of 3® members some ideas! It's amazing to me how many people routinely say, "I don't know what to say to say 'I love you.'" Uh—how about saying "I love you"? Ideas about acts of loving-kindness to children, colleagues, friends, parents, other family members are always welcome. Ideas about how to show loving-kindness to enemies or adversaries can be life changing and enormously beneficial.

On our Web site, we provide a place to journal TOP 1™ actions.

If you sense that a team partner is striving for beauty, striving for perfection, or is hungry for acceptance, offer extra affirmations to that person about his or her character traits or behaviors that you admire. Let the person know that you value him or her solely as your faithful team partner.

SPEAKING DICTUMS FOR EMOTIONAL FITNESS

The dictums related to emotional fitness are an important way of taking charge over what you *choose* to do and be. Choose a set of dictums that speak to having love, joy, and peace as the dominant emotional traits of your life. You can address other emotions in your dictums, but generally speaking, all dictums aimed at emotional fitness are likely to be linked to love, joy, and peace in some way. For example, if you desire to have greater patience in your life, that certainly is linked to greater peace. If you desire to be less prejudiced toward others, that likely is to be linked to love.

The more you recognize a lack of a particular emotional trait in your life, the more important it is to speak your dictums with strength. You may benefit greatly by speaking these dictums repeatedly throughout a day. Several people have told me that they command themselves in each of these areas of love, joy, and peace several times a day. Do what works for you.

Possible Emotional Fitness Dictums

1. I AM joyful.
2. I AM faithful.
3. I AM a peacemaker.
4. I AM thankful.
5. I AM valuable.
6. I AM loving.
7. I AM putting others first.

COACH'S CLIPBOARD

I'm a coach, and coaches give their players specific exercises as a part of workout drills. So . . . here are your exercises for this chapter!

Check your emotions.

Exercise: Evaluate your own thinking and feeling about "fading beauty," "perfectionism," and your "hunger level for acceptance." Are there emotional fitness goals you need to make with regard to these three issues?

Choose or refuse.

Exercise: Love, joy, and peace are healthy and balanced emotions. What do you need to refuse or choose to build more of each into your life?

To experience more love:	☐ I choose	☐ I refuse
To experience more joy:	☐ I choose	☐ I refuse
To experience more peace:	☐ I choose	☐ I refuse

Set your goals and get started.

Exercise: Using the Choose/Refuse answers above, lay out your ten-week goals to increase your emotional fitness.

Exercise: Write out your own emotional fitness dictums. Begin to speak them daily.

Put the other person first.
Exercise: Identify a set of people to bless with at least two TOP 1™ deeds each.

Be accountable to others.
Exercise: Report daily to your Team of 3® on your TOP 1™ activity.

TOTALLY FIT LIFE TRUTH

The feelings we express are the feelings that others will hold toward us. What we do and say to others become what others do and say to us.

CHAPTER 9

You Are What You Think:
Mental Fitness After 40

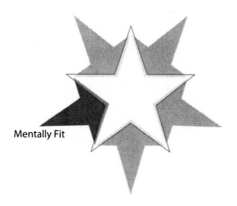

Mentally Fit

I am convinced that the saying "You are what you eat" is true. I am equally convinced that "You are what you *think*" is true.

Pat was certainly an example of this to me. She came to the Totally Fit Life program several years ago at the age of forty-nine. Her fiftieth birthday was about to be her magical milestone birthday. Pat's husband had died eighteen years before she arrived at our program—and she was still in deep grief. The sorrow Pat felt about losing her husband in a plane crash had clouded her every decision and relationship. She admitted to me, "I think about him all the time."

"How many times a day do you think about Gene?" I asked.

"Probably a hundred times."

"What specifically do you think about?" I asked.

"Everything. Things we did. Things he said. What he would probably be doing today. What he would probably say in different situations. How he looked. What he liked and didn't like. Everything."

Pat had decorated her condo the way Gene would have liked it—not necessarily in her own style. She dressed in the way she knew Gene would have liked, which wasn't all that fashionable today. She stored up tidbits of information each day to tell Gene in nightly conversations she had with him. She was living a significant part of each day in a world, and in a relationship, that wasn't in this present reality. When it came to mental fitness, Pat had some serious work to do if she was going to be "whole" for the remainder of her life.

Mental fitness has a number of facets to it, all of which seem to be increasingly important after the age of forty. These five facets of mental fitness can be summed up in one definitive statement: *Mental fitness is clear thinking in the present moment, with good memories and good values upon which to draw for creative solutions; an ability to make sound decisions; and a strong will to continue generating new ideas and complete beneficial work.*

MENTAL KEENNESS

Mental keenness includes several mental abilities: the ability to attend to (perceive), focus on (concentrate), and remember various stimuli. These are characteristics that health-care experts often focus on as they diagnose dementia of various types. The goal of healthy mental function is to be able to perceive things accurately, have the ability to focus and retain focus upon a particular thought or concept, and have the ability to remember important facts and concepts.

Perception

Perhaps the single most important aspect of staying mentally sharp involves a person's ability to pay attention. Your mind must be alert and ready to receive information. At times you may need to tell yourself to *wake up!* That's another way of saying, *Get in the present moment!* Don't dwell on memories or daydreams to the point that you miss what's happening around you. At times you may need to tell yourself to *pay attention!* The more stimuli in any given moment, the more you have to force yourself to remain alert to what is happening all around you.

There are a number of things that can cloud perception, as well as the ability to concentrate or remember. These include preconceptions or prejudices. Midlife is a good time to evaluate why you may not like certain classes of people or why you think certain things need to be done in certain ways.

Stress can cloud perception—especially stress that arises from taking on too many responsibilities and tasks in too limited a time frame, with too great an expectation of perfection. A person with a massive deadline or an overwhelming problem often has difficulty seeing the "new thing" or even the "right solution."

Medications can cloud perception, and so can poor nutrition—too much sugar, for example, can create a "sugar low" that literally causes some people to "zone out." Being perceptive to detail is nearly impossible if the brain is fuzzed out on drugs, including sugar.

Concentration

Concentration is the ability to focus and then sustain focus. Many people struggle with this in midlife and after. This may actually be the result of people acquiring so many rote habits and learned skills; they may not be facing very many new tasks or challenges that require them to focus in order to learn. Concentration is necessary for a good memory. The less time a person spends concentrating on something, the less likely that information is going to be stored for long-term retrieval.

Memory

Some memory loss is benign. Don't panic if you have minor lapses of memory or find yourself searching for a word or name. Brief momentary lapses can occur at any age. Also, some information isn't worth remembering. You probably don't need to remember, for example, the phone number you had when you were a freshman in college.

You need to be concerned, however, if your memory loss results in a period of confusion over what time it is or where you are, if people point out that you are asking the same questions or making the same statements repeatedly in a short period of time, if you get lost while driving a route that is familiar to you, completely forget an appointment with someone important to you, are unable to remember how to conduct simple transactions such as writing a check, or have difficulty in naming very familiar objects. If these memory problems arise, seek professional help.

Now that we've covered the waterfront of mental acuity in a very broad overview, let's focus on the practical things you can do to stay alert:

Keep reading and writing. Read a variety of materials, both nonfiction and fiction.

Work mental and word puzzles. Work a variety of puzzles, such as logic, crossword, and word puzzles, as well as difficult jigsaw puzzles.

Have a real conversation with someone. Turn off the television and radio.

Cross-train your brain. Make up songs, sing or stay active in some form of musical expression, including memorization of song lyrics. Take an art class and seek to do things "artistically." Read poetry aloud; memorize poetic passages you find amusing or meaningful. These activities help keep the left and right sides of the brain in balance. One of the things medical researchers have discovered is that in the aftermath of a stroke, the "other" side of the brain not affected by the stroke has an amazing ability to compensate for the damaged brain tissue. The more balanced the overall brain function had been prior to the stroke, the more this ability is enhanced.

Another aspect of cross-training is to seek to learn in a way that isn't normally your style. People tend to be visual learners (what they see), kinesthetic learners (what they do, or movement of some type), or auditory learners (what they hear). Try learning new things in a new way.

Build your vocabulary. Look up words you don't know and begin to use them.

Organize memorabilia so that you can readily access the objects associated with events in the past. You'll be able to recall greater detail about a person or experience if you can see and touch items related to the memory you are seeking to access.

Work on memory-related puzzles. Some of these are available at various Internet sites. The more you develop strong memory skills now, the better your memory is likely to be in the years ahead.

And above all:

Learn something new. The more you keep learning and exploring the world around you, the healthier your mental function will be. Keep growing intellectually. Perhaps take a course in an area you have been interested in but have never formally studied. Consider taking a course that requires a certain amount of creativity.

GOOD DECISION MAKING

Good mental acuity is necessary for making good decisions, including the setting of goals. The setting of a goal always begins with what you believe is possible. I often ask the people who sign up for the Totally Fit Life program, "What do you think you can do?" It is far more productive to focus on what you think you can do, rather than what you think you can't do. It is also far more challenging to focus on what you *think* you can do, generally with a little effort, planning, or practice, rather than on what you actually can do at any given time.

You may want to pause for a moment and look back over some of the goals you have written down for your first ten-week cycle in the areas of fitness we have already covered. Have you set your goals high enough? Will they truly challenge what you *think* you can do?

I have talked to lots of people through the years who needed to lose fifty pounds of fat but didn't believe they could—so they haven't. I've also talked to people who needed to lose that much fat and more and believed they could do it with some encouragement and effort—and they did.

I have talked to lots of people who never thought they could climb out of the general depression or feelings that they were experiencing—and they didn't, in spite of people encouraging them almost around the clock. I've also talked to people who were very depressed, and for good cause, who believed that tomorrow might be brighter. And while it didn't happen overnight for some of these people, the days did eventually get brighter. They can hardly believe now that they were once on the borderline of being clinically depressed.

What you think about long enough, even what you hold as a subliminal thought, is eventually what you do. That's been proven in countless studies. Your thoughts—call them dreams, hopes—give rise to certain attitudes and thought patterns that give you an automatic bent toward certain types of information, stimuli, and situations. You begin to feel drawn to various people and experiences. And eventually, you participate in those experiences or enter those relationships. The more you do so, the more your behavior becomes fixed—even habitual.

This can work for good or bad, of course. If you are fantasizing about bad behavior with the wrong crowd, you can soon find yourself engaged in bad behavior with the wrong crowd. If, on the other hand, you are fantasizing about doing great and noble things with godly people, you very likely will find yourself engaged in good behaviors with good people—and sooner rather than later.

Some people criticize imagination. I thank God for it. Our ability to imagine has been given to us so that we can begin to "see" and believe for good things to come. Our imaginations help set our thinking in a direction, and as long as that direction is positive and rooted in godly values, imagination can be a tremendous asset. In some cases, you may be wise to ask yourself, *What do I believe might be done?* Some people who don't believe something *can* be done at present are quick to say that something *might* be done in the future. If "might be done" is all you can muster up—go for it. The "can be done" will come in good time.

Check your thought life. What you are believing for, what you think you can do or would like to do, and what you imagine as a possibility will set the foundation for your decision making.

DEALING WITH PAINFUL MEMORIES

Back to Pat, whom I mentioned in the beginning of this chapter; Pat's main difficulty in achieving true mental fitness was in learning to let go of the painful past and live in a hopeful present. There are two words in that previous sentence that are very important.

Pat needed to *learn* to let go of the past. The mind has habits that are just as deeply ingrained, and perhaps more so, than physical habits or addictions. Learning to change your thought processes is one of the most important things you can ever learn to do. As I began to challenge

Pat about her constant obsession with thoughts of Gene, she said: "I don't think I can stop thinking about Gene."

I said, "It probably will be very difficult, Pat. You've been thinking about him night and day for eighteen years, and in your marriage, much longer than eighteen years. The real question you need to ask yourself is, *Do I want to think about him less often?*"

"Well, you and other people tell me I need to think about him less often. I don't really *want* to quit thinking about him, but I suppose I *need* to think about him less often," Pat said.

"Keep in mind, Pat," I said, "that your family members and close friends are not asking you to stop thinking about Gene altogether. Neither am I. We just want you to be able to think about other things and remain a productive, creative person who is also devoting some mental energy to making a difference in the world around you."

"I want that," Pat said. "I do want to be productive, creative, and make a difference."

We started at that point. We focused on goals that Pat still had for her life. We spent considerable time discussing her directional goals as well as her emotional goals.

I asked, "What kind of *thinking* do you need to do to accomplish each of these goals?" We took the goals one by one. In some cases, Pat said she felt that she needed to learn a new skill or acquire new information. In some cases, she felt that she needed to immerse herself totally in a project—in something that took her full concentration.

Pat identified several people whom she wanted to bless with a TOP 1™ deed every day. One of those people was her granddaughter Irene. Another was a friend of Irene's who had lost both of her parents in an automobile accident. We talked about the need for Pat to work hard on listening skills and to become creative in planning special outings and experiences for Irene and her friend Marcy.

A very specific thing Pat and I concluded that she needed to address was her "talking things over with Gene" each night. The solution to that was for Pat to seek out other friends whom she could talk to. Over several months, Pat did develop two close friends. She called one her "fun" friend. Pat delighted in telling amusing experiences and outlandish adventures to her. The other friend she called her "serious" friend. Pat felt totally free to talk to this friend about serious, sad, and spiritual experiences. Pat made two other new friends: her Team of 3® partners! Both of these friends were also recovering from losses, and they not only had special insight into what Pat was going through but also offered some helpful suggestions.

I learned a great deal in my work with Pat. I came away with three strong conclusions about how to change mental patterns that are painful—especially those rooted in grief over the loss of a loved one and sorrow over what was lost as the result of abuse or rejection.

First, it is vitally important in changing a mental habit that you find something to *give* that requires your full attention. When you get involved in an activity that demands your mental and emotional focus, you have less time to dwell on what has been painful in the past.

Second, it is important to have friends or counselors with whom you can talk over the processes of loss and recovery. It is especially important to have a counselor who has the same values that you have, and who has your best interests at heart. It is crucial to have someone to talk to who has been through at least a little bit of what you have experienced.

Third, it is important that you choose to forgive. To forgive is to "let go." It is not the same as exoneration, and it certainly is not denial. Forgiveness is *not* saying that something didn't hurt or doesn't deserve to be addressed with justice. It is saying, *I won't be bound to this.* In Pat's case, she came to a point where she truly needed to forgive Gene for leaving her—for taking that business trip in that particular airplane on that particular day. She knew objectively that Gene hadn't purposefully left her or made a decision to die. Emotionally, however, and subliminally in her thoughts, she was holding on to the idea that if Gene hadn't gone on the trip, he'd be alive today.

She needed to let go of all blame. In a rather mystical way, she needed to "let Gene die." She said, "Coach, I needed to let Gene go to heaven. I needed to begin to see him *there*, not *here*. I needed to begin to trust that he was fully alive and well and would be waiting for me in the future, rather than hang on to trying to keep him alive and waiting for me at the end of every day."

Get involved in giving.

Stay in communication with loving friends who are good at listening to your pain and encouraging you to move forward.

Forgive, and then forgive some more.

A STOREHOUSE OF GOOD IDEAS

Mental fitness always involves having *good* things to think about. It's the same as with nutritional issues we addressed in chapter 7. You need to have *good* things to think about with *good* frequency in *good* amounts!

Just as with your physical body—garbage in, garbage out. A highly negative attitude will overtake you if you routinely choose to think about things that you know are wrong, sinful, manipulative, dishonest, untrue, lustful, hate-filled, greed-focused, or mean-spirited. Such an attitude is totally opposite what it takes to reach positive goals or to enjoy a Totally Fit Life.

Choose to think about what is good, noble, positive, pleasant, and pure, not the ugly gossip or horror stories that spread so easily in our conversations.

Choose to think about what you want to remember five years from now, ten years from now, or longer into the future. To make good memories, think good thoughts and then act on them.

MAINTAINING A WILL
TO LIVE A HIGH-QUALITY LIFE

Part of living a Totally Fit Life for the rest of your life means having a strong will to live a high-quality life for as long as possible, so that you might accomplish as much of your God-given purpose on this earth as you can. If you are in the habit of saying *I will* statements to yourself, you are much more likely to command yourself with *I will* commands should you become seriously ill or injured, or should you suffer a major setback or loss.

"*I will* rebuild."
"*I will* love again."
"*I will* get well."
"*I will* get out of bed and face the day."
"*I will* do my physical rehabilitation exercises."
"*I will* succeed this time."
"*I will* fill out one more application."
"*I will* pay off this debt."
"*I will* choose to hope."
"*I will* get to church this morning."

I recently heard about a woman who was badly injured in a motorcycle accident who said through tears each morning: "*I will* get out of this bed and walk down to the nursing station."

The first three days she made it only part of the way, each day getting a little bit closer to the nursing station before she had to sit down or return to her room. The fourth day she made her goal! This was an important milestone for her, but it certainly wasn't her "big goal." She was walking with the aid of a walker when she first went to the nursing station. Her big goal was to walk unaided across an auditorium platform to receive a major award she was scheduled to receive in six weeks. Her *I will* attitude and statements got her to that awards platform on time.

Beyond Emotion

The speaking of *I will* statements moves a person beyond a negative emotion and also beyond an "I don't feel like it today" attitude. A person who is dependent upon how he or she feels is going to be a person who is always looking for excuses. Don't get stuck in your feelings. Move into your *will.*

I will statements are particularly effective in helping you get through those times of tension, frustration, and friction that are a normal part of growth and change. We all like the idea of having grown and changed for the better. I don't know anybody, however, who actually enjoys the pain and frustration of making changes and experiencing growing pains. (They are called growing *pains* for a reason!)

Keeping your will active and vibrant will help you get through times of frustration until a new and healthy habit is fully in place. How long do you need to continue to speak *I will* statements related to the specific behaviors linked to your goals? Oh—at least ten weeks.

ESTABLISHING GOALS FOR MENTAL FITNESS

As is true for each area of the Totally Fit Life, your goals are *your* goals. What is it that you intuitively know that you need to change about your thought patterns in order to accomplish the following?

- Think more clearly (with greater mental keenness) in the present moment
- Develop good memories and establish good values

- Be more creative in problem solving
- Make wise judgments and choices
- Promote the development of a strong, faith-based will

Write down your goals. Then write down *I will* statements associated with various behaviors that are a natural part of pursuing, accomplishing, or maintaining each goal.

MENTAL FITNESS AND YOUR TEAM OF 3®

When it comes to your specific accountability to your Team of 3® in this area, you need to discuss how you want to self-report progress toward goals you each have set for mental growth.

You may want the accountability to be very simple:

Learned something new:	☐ yes	☐ no
Willed myself to succeed:	☐ yes	☐ no
Had a good thought life:	☐ yes	☐ no

You intuitively know if you learned something, used *I will* statements to good advantage, and had a pure, good, virtuous thought life on any given day. You intuitively know if you spoke positively about yourself during the day, or if you didn't.

You may want the accountability to be more precise. If so, make sure that your other Team of 3® members also want that degree of precision in their reporting back to you.

If you notice that you are routinely or frequently saying no in reporting on mental fitness criteria to your Team of 3®, you may want to talk to your team members about the difficulty you are having. Ask them for *positive* input. If you notice that another team member is routinely reporting no, you may want to ask if the person is having a problem with a particular mental fitness goal. Be willing to listen, and if you have something positive to offer to the person, share it. Do not, however, use these times for gossiping about other people, tearing down other people, or justifying a negative attitude or thought process. Mutually agree that you will help one another think positively in order to build a more positive life.

Choose to be especially positive in talking about your ideas and thoughts about fitness, nutrition, emotional well-being, faith, learning or education, wholeness, goal making, and so forth. Any time you begin to criticize something, you lessen the likelihood that you will achieve the goals that you believe—or once believed—were worthy to pursue.

SPEAKING DICTUMS FOR MENTAL FITNESS

The dictums below are offered to give you some sample ideas as you begin to establish your own dictums related to your mental fitness. They are dictums that envision the reality that you *are* mentally fit! Write down your own dictums and begin to speak them with firm conviction.

Possible Mental Fitness Dictums
1. I AM thinking pure thoughts.
2. I AM taking charge of my thought life.
3. I AM thinking about solutions.
4. I AM thinking noble thoughts.
5. I AM speaking positively.
6. I AM learning something new.
7. I AM memorizing inspirational phrases.

COACH'S CLIPBOARD

I'm a coach, and coaches give their players specific exercises as a part of workout drills. So . . . here are your exercises for this chapter!

Set your course.

Exercise: Set specific ten-week goals to improve your:

- Perception ability

- Concentration ability

- Memory

You're never too old to learn.

Exercise: Identify three things you'd like to learn, or learn "better," or learn in a new way (with a different learning style).

175

The will to win.

Exercise: Make a list of "I WILL" statements to go along with various goals you have set in other areas of the Fitness Star. Remember that these statements relate to *behavior.*

Character counts.

Exercise: Write out a set of "I AM" dictums—aimed at *character*—for mental fitness and begin to voice them to yourself daily.

Be accountable to others.

Exercise: Report daily to your Team of 3® on your progress in pursuit of your mental fitness goals.

TOTALLY FIT LIFE TRUTH

Choose your thoughts wisely.
They guide what you do.
They become who you are.

CHAPTER 10

Radiating Life from Core Values:
Spiritual Fitness After 40

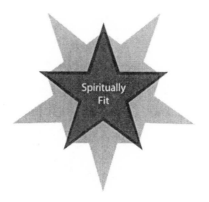

Fitness also has a spiritual dimension. As I stated in an earlier chapter, spiritual fitness is at the *center* of the Totally Fit Life program. Why? Because ultimately what a person believes about God, the relationship between God and man, and the relationship God desires for people to have with one another are all directly linked to a person's emotional, mental, and directional fitness. And it is what a person establishes as goals in the emotional, mental, and directional fitness areas that impact greatly what a person sets as physical and nutritional fitness goals. Let me illustrate.

John came to the program when he was forty-five. That was his magical milestone birthday. He complained that in his work as an international salesman in an energy-related industry he tended to put on weight when he was traveling, which was often for two to three weeks at a time across many time zones. He said, "I've always been able to lose those excess pounds after a few days back in the gym, but not any longer. My body just doesn't cooperate like it once did. I need to get more fit."

I explained to John that the Totally Fit Life program was about far more than physical fitness. John seemed ready for the totality of what the program offers. He readily admitted that he had some nutritional fitness issues, and that there were some areas of intellectual and emotional fitness he'd be willing to address. He seemed almost eager to get into directional fitness goal setting. Then I asked him how he felt about spiritual fitness goals. At that, John balked a little.

"I've never been much on church," he said. "I know you are a Christian. You've been upfront about that, and I respect your faith. But as for me— well, I suppose I'd put down *Christian* on a hospital form that might ask me to identify a particular faith, but I haven't been to church since I was about six years old. Church just hasn't been a priority."

"This program isn't about church," I said. "Spiritual fitness addresses some very basic beliefs." I went on to explain that spiritual fitness starts with three sets of questions:

1. What do you believe about your reason for being on this earth? Is it a random accident without purpose, or do you believe that you were divinely created for a purpose? The answer obviously relates to the overall directional fitness goals you are going to set for yourself. The basic reason to be as healthy as possible, which is

directly related to physical and nutritional fitness, is to live as high a quality of life as possible for as long as possible to fulfill as much of your reason for living as possible. If a person doesn't have a reason for living, it is likely that person is going to have a much lower expectation about how whole or healthy he or she can be or should be.

2. Do you believe God desires to have a relationship with you? And do you desire to be in relationship with God? If you don't believe God can have—or desires to have—a personal relationship with you, is there part of you that wishes it *might* be possible? Would you like to know that God is on your side? The answers go straight to the heart of motivation. Do you live solely to please yourself, or do you live to please your Creator? Do you behave in ways that are totally self-focused, or do you behave in ways that are in obedience to the commands and desires of One greater than you?

3. How do you believe that human beings were designed to live in relationship with one another? Obviously men and women were designed to produce babies, which means that from the beginning of the human race, people were intended to live in families and extended families (tribes) and communities. What are the rules and principles that govern those relationships?

John, who was something of a tough guy in the way he appeared and acted on the exterior, surprised me with his answer. "I think it all comes down to love," he said. "The reason I'm here on earth is to love somebody—maybe a few people, maybe even more than a few people. I believe in love."

"Love is your basic value for life?" I asked.

"Yeah, I guess so," John said.

"Let's start there, then," I said. "Loving is the main spiritual fitness value that you have."

I then showed John this basic definition of spiritual fitness:

Identifying your core values and the reason you hold them, so you might build upon them and express them as fully as possible.

Your first challenge when it comes to spiritual fitness is to identify your core values. I suspect they won't be all that different from the ones John identified.

LOVING OTHERS

For most people, having somebody to love is a very good reason to get up each morning! Love of family, especially, seems to be a very big part of the identity most people have. It's a core value. How fit are you when it comes to loving your family members and friends?

Being spiritually fit means that you have the energy, capacity, and desire to express your values to other people. When it comes to love, you need to *have* love to be able to *give* love. If you aren't receiving enough love in your life, what might you do to give more love? To whom might you give more love, and in what appropriate ways?

You need to be intentional in seeking out times and ways in which to express love. Love doesn't just "happen." It isn't just floating around in the air like some mystical allergen waiting to be inhaled by somebody's heart. It must be planted, cultivated, and nurtured between people.

As you begin to anticipate your spiritual fitness goals, pay special attention to ways in which you might better develop genuinely loving relationships with others.

A word of caution: Don't confuse lust and love. Don't confuse flirtation with love. Genuine love has a depth and purity that go far beyond sexual attraction, and even far beyond "being nice" to a friend or family member.

Genuine love has a sacrificial quality to it. A person who loves is willing to give, even if that giving costs time, energy, talent, or resources. Genuine love involves giving even when giving is inconvenient and is not reciprocated.

Forgiveness

One of the foremost displays of genuine love is forgiveness. Note that the word *give* is at the heart of forgiveness. For*give*ness is truly a gift that we give to one another. It is setting the person who hurt you free from the prison cell of your heart where you have been holding him or her so that you can exact justice for the pain you've felt. When you release that person to "go free," you are also set free! You no longer need to fear being in the presence of the person. You no longer are tied up emotionally by feelings of bitterness, anger, or resentment.

Be quick to forgive. It's the most loving thing you can do.

"But what," Ron asked me, "if the person you are forgiving doesn't receive your forgiveness—or even think that they need your forgiveness?"

It doesn't matter whether another person asks for your forgiveness. Forgive anyway. Forgiveness happens in your heart. Say aloud to the vacant air if you need to: "I forgive you"—and name the person by name. Release that person from your heart. The person may never know that you have done this, but I can guarantee you that if you have genuinely set the person free, he or she will intuitively sense that freedom the next time he or she is around you.

The person you have forgiven will no longer feel constrained, manipulated, criticized, or tied to you. It's a great mystery how this happens, but I know it does happen. He or she may be surprised and may even conclude that you don't care. In truth, you have cared enough to do the most loving thing you can do—to give that person the freedom to judge him- or herself.

In the same way, if somebody comes to you and asks for forgiveness, be quick to give it! You may not have even realized there was a problem.

Don't try to justify your behavior or point out additional faults with the other person. Give forgiveness quickly, freely, and fully.

If somebody comes to tell you that you have hurt or wronged him or her, don't argue or try to justify your behavior. Simply ask that person what you might do to make amends, say you are sorry, and ask the person to forgive you. It doesn't matter who is right. It matters that you live in peace and forgiveness with each other.

Living in a forgiven state with other people, and especially with those who live in close contact with you daily, is vital for both spiritual and emotional fitness. Don't trespass against others. In other words, don't trample on their personal or emotional turf—and don't hold the trespasses of others against them. Jesus taught this at the heart of His teaching on prayer: "Forgive us our debts, as we forgive our debtors" (Matthew 6:12 NKJV).

As you explore spiritual fitness goals, identify people you may need to forgive—both for their sakes and your sake. If you need to go to someone to ask for forgiveness, make a specific plan to do so.

Role-Modeling Love

I have a very strong awareness every day that I am a role model to my three children. I take that responsibility very seriously. Although my wife is certainly not required in any way to follow my example, I am aware that she is greatly influenced by the way I speak and act, just as I am greatly influenced by the way she speaks and acts. I seek daily to live in a *loving* relationship with my wife and children. I want love to flow freely in our home, and I want my children to extend the love of our family to their friends, and one day, to their own spouses. What we model to one another in our family, we seek to model in our church and community.

Love is expressed primarily by presence (being there for others, especially in crisis times); tangible gifts (related to needs or simply generous expressions of affection); words (there's no substitute for saying "I love you" often and with heartfelt sincerity); and physical affection (hugs and kisses, pats on the shoulder, and so forth—whatever is appropriate for the relationship). Sometimes just reaching out to a person in a letter or phone call can be an expression of love. The point is to express love to other people in ways that they can receive it and desire it. Do what is meaningful to the other person, not just what seems convenient, easy, or meaningful to you. That's what giving is all about.

As you establish your spiritual fitness goals, identify ways in which you might teach others to love by example, not just by word. Showing someone else how to give and receive love is far more potent than merely telling another person to be more loving. Also identify ways in which you might better express love to specific people.

LOVING SELF

As indicated earlier, it's impossible to give great love if you do not have a reservoir of love in your heart from which to draw. It is always possible, however, to give *some* love. Start with what you have to give, and work on building up a large reservoir of love in your heart so that you can give more and more love as the weeks, months, and years unfold before you.

How do you "get" love? Start giving—to somebody. I recommend children in need. They nearly always respond quickly and generously to pure expressions of love from others. Soak up their hugs and their delight in being with you. Older people in need also are worthy of your expressions of love. Give generously to them, without any thought of what you might get back. You'll *feel* love in return as you recognize how much you are brightening their day and making them feel valuable and worthy.

Become a little introspective about the way you feel about your own life. We touched on this in the chapter on emotional fitness. Go deeper at this time. Do you see anything in your life that keeps you from being lovable?

Many people are shackled by feelings of guilt and shame. Guilt comes when we know we have done something wrong. Shame comes when we know something wrong has been done to us, and we are the innocent victims or unwilling partners in the wrong behavior. Both guilt and shame are erased by forgiveness. As a Christian, I draw upon God's free offer of forgiveness as my starting point in forgiving myself.

If I need to ask forgiveness of another person, that's also an important step in my being set free from guilt. If I am feeling shame for something that happened to me, then I need to forgive the person who put me in that position of shame. Finally, I recognize that I need to forgive myself—I need to quit rehearsing the "what ifs" and "whys" of past wrong behavior and move on with my life. I need to set my own mind and heart free from the hurtful memories and feelings.

It's very difficult to love yourself if you are still blaming yourself, continuing to see yourself as a person unworthy of love, or reeling from the blunt-force pain of open rejection. Ask God to restore to you a deep sense of your own identity. Seek forgiveness and then freely forgive yourself!

LOVING GOD

As a Christian, part of my spiritual fitness core is a deep love for God. Having a personal relationship with God is vital to my life. I don't know how to feel fully forgiven and cleansed of all sin, guilt, and shame, apart from having a relationship with God. Everything about my reason for being, and the ways in which I choose to live in relationship with other people, is linked in some way to my relationship with God and His commandments over my life.

How does a person show love to an invisible, awesome, infinite God? First, by obeying Him. That's the number one criterion offered by the

Bible. Jesus even said to His followers: "If you love Me, you will obey what I have told you to do" (see John 14:15–23).

We love God by obeying His commandments about our behavior and also by following His prescribed methods, including the method God prescribed for the full forgiveness of our sins—receiving Jesus Christ as our Savior and then seeking to follow Him as our Lord. The most famous verse in the New Testament says, "For God so loved the world that He gave His only begotten Son, that whoever believes in Him should not perish but have everlasting life" (John 3:16 NKJV). God's promise is that when we believe that Jesus is the Savior, we experience full forgiveness of our sins, come into a full and loving personal relationship with our Creator, and receive His gift of eternal life.

One of the primary ways that we obey God is by seeking to fulfill the purpose He had in mind when He created us. We need to find our purpose and pursue it—that's what directional fitness is all about. We obey God when we identify our talents, develop skills that improve our talents, and then give those talents away to people in need. We obey God when we encourage others to do likewise.

Second, we express love to God by *giving* to Him. What can we give to God? Our devotion, our trust, our loyalty, our time and presence in prayer, our expressions of praise and thanksgiving. We can give our resources toward efforts that promote God's plan and purposes on this earth—not only His plan for forgiveness but also His plans for caring for the needs of His people.

Many people seem to see obedience as difficult and service to God as drudgery. They see giving to the Lord, including those aspects of giving that are spiritual disciplines, as obligations that diminish a person's resources and identity. I see these things in just the opposite light. God's commandments are for our benefit, not only in eternity but right now. If every person kept the Ten Commandments, this world would not be more boring or less creative. It would be much more exciting and much more loving, joyful, peaceable, creative, and energetic! It would be a world with much less stress, heartache, and suffering. It would be much less like hell and much more like heaven!

Giving to the Lord—of *anything* that is good, and with a cheerful attitude—always reaps a tremendous harvest much greater than what is given. That is a universal principle throughout the New Testament. Jesus said, "Give, and it will be given to you: good measure, pressed down, shaken together, and running over will be put into your bosom. For with the same measure that you use, it will be measured back to you" (Luke 6:38 NKJV).

Every seed that is planted and grows on this earth produces a harvest of seeds that is greater than the seed planted. That's a basic law of nature. The greater harvest is promised for the good that we plant into our world. The New Testament also says, "Let us not grow weary while doing good, for in due season we shall reap if we do not lose heart" (Galatians 6:9 NKJV).

Part of our giving to God is giving to God our lives in a sacrificial way—that He might "use" us in any way He desires. The apostle Paul wrote to the early Christian church in Rome about this. He said, "I beseech you therefore, brethren, by the mercies of God, that you present your bodies a living sacrifice, holy, acceptable to God, which is your reasonable service" (Romans 12:1 NKJV). One of my personal spiritual fitness goals is to present to God the "sharpest" Don Nava that I can give to Him, so God can use me to the max.

I'm not a woodworker, but I have friends who are. They tell me that they spend as much time sharpening and caring for the tools in their workshops as they do in making things. They must have tools that are in good condition. Saws and axes need to be sharp, tools with handles and moving parts need to be fitted together tightly, tools with motors and engines need to be well fueled and lubricated, and so forth. I strongly believe that each person is a tool of some kind in God's hands. We need to do our part to keep ourselves in the best working order possible, and trust God to sharpen us, refine us, and use us as He desires.

If loving God is part of how you define spiritual fitness, I strongly encourage you to consider spiritual fitness goals that are aimed at greater obedience to God's commandments and greater giving to God.

OTHER SPIRITUAL QUALITIES THAT ARE PART OF SPIRITUAL FITNESS

There are other spiritual aspects that are certainly part of spiritual fitness: purity, faith, potential, creativity, and wisdom. You may want to consider these qualities of your spiritual life and can begin now to work on your own definition of a spiritually fit life with a look at these first two aspects.

Purity

The Totally Fit Life calls for purity in every area of life. Physical exercise purifies the body by helping to eliminate toxins and stress; eating pure foods and drinking pure water are key factors in nutritional fitness; thinking pure thoughts contributes to mental fitness; rooting relationships in purity is vital for emotional fitness; and pursuing "pure" goals gives life greater direction and meaning.

The spiritual life is also marked to some degree by purity. Many religions have rituals related to cleansing—fasting, washing, bathing, baptizing, and so forth. Many religions call for a purifying of the mind and soul, with various rituals associated with purification. There's a link between what we do to cleanse the body and mind and what God does to cleanse the spirit. I encourage you, as an act of spiritual fitness, to ask yourself these four questions about purity:

1. Am I taking into my system—body, mind, and spirit—things that contribute to purity?
2. Am I routinely engaging in habits that contribute to purity of the world around me?
3. Am I responding to life and setting goals that reflect a purity of motivation and a purity of character?
4. Am I seeking to build relationships that are pure—innocent of immorality or illegality, and free of manipulation and hurtful behavior?

Faith

Every religion is in some way rooted in belief. What a person believes about God, self, other people, and ways of relating to God are at the heart of every religion. In addition, every religion requires its adherents to put their beliefs into action. Some kind of application of faith and values is expected when it comes to what a person thinks, says, and does. There are two questions that I hope you will consider as you weigh various aspects of spiritual fitness in your life.

1. Do you believe God desires for you to be totally fit?
2. Do you believe God will help you to become more fit and to live a Totally Fit Life?

Certainly my answer to both of these questions is a resounding *yes!*

Greg asked me, "How do I ask God to help me achieve my Totally Fit Life goals?"

I said, "Use these four words: *God, please help me.*" I have absolutely no doubt that if a person speaks those words to God with sincerity of heart and a true desire to do what contributes to wholeness, God will give His help!

Many people through the years have greatly benefited by praying very specifically for God's help as they pursue goals in various areas of the Totally Fit Life program:

"God, please help me to eat the right things today."

"God, please help me to awaken early tomorrow morning feeling rested and ready to go to the gym to work out."

"God, please help me to think the right thoughts."

"God, please help me to respond to other people today as You desire for me to respond to them—with love and forgiveness."

I find in my own life that when I combine my prayer petitions to God with *I will* statements, I have much stronger willpower. God supplies His power to my will—and that is the most potent form of willpower I know!

LINKING YOUR WILL TO YOUR FAITH

I have met many people through the years—mostly in Christian circles—who see their will and their faith as conflicting. They believe that if they "will" to do something, they are not trusting God enough. Others believe that they have no right to trust God to do all the work in their lives. They usually say such things as, "God gave me a good mind and a healthy body, and He expects me to use them."

I don't see a conflict between will and faith. I believe they were designed to work together. When I voice *I will* statements, I usually say, "with God's help." At other times, I know that "with God's help" is a firm pillar of my attitude, and that even if I say *I will,* I am truly believing that what I'm about to do is a part of God's will for me, and therefore, God will help me accomplish what I am setting myself to do.

It seems the key is knowing that what you are choosing to do is also what God has chosen for you. If you are a Christian, does God desire for you to be a person who is a witness to the love and saving grace of Jesus? Absolutely. If you choose to speak the name of Jesus to a person who doesn't know Jesus, or to a person who needs to be reminded of Jesus' love and power to heal, deliver, reconcile, and save—God certainly has chosen that for you!

Does God desire for you to be a person who is loving, joyful, peace-loving, longsuffering, kind, good, faithful, gentle, and in self-control of his own tongue and body? Absolutely. He said as much, calling these the "fruit" of the Holy Spirit's work in the life of a Christian! (see Galatians 5:22–23). If you choose to do a loving deed, speak joyful praise and thanksgiving, or engage in a gentle expression of God's compassion—God certainly has chosen that for you!

I can say with great confidence:

- *I will* read a chapter of the New Testament. (I know God is in full favor of my doing that.)
- *I will* take captive every stray thought as I read God's Word. (Certainly that is fully in keeping with God's desire for me.)
- *I will* pray for each of my family members. (God desires for me to do that, and I believe that as I pray, He may very well bring other concerns to my mind so that I can pray about them during my prayer time.)
- *I will* treat each person I encounter with the utmost respect and love. (God desires this for me in all of my relationships, even with strangers or those who may not have my best interests at heart.)
- *I will* be sensitive to the leading of God during this upcoming business appointment. (Does God desire for me to trust Him in all things—all decisions, all choices, all conversations, all business transactions? I believe He does! I can say *I will* with great confidence.)

There are countless things I can say *I will* about, knowing with the full confidence of faith that God's promise to me is "Amen" to that action or the development of that character trait in my life. Even as I say *I will*, I am also trusting God to help me *do* what it is I am willing to do. I am trusting that God will use me as His willing servant in every situation, even as I trust God to do His good and perfecting work in me through the words and deeds of other people.

Will and faith are definitely linked any time we say, "*I will* believe God" or "*I will* trust God." When it comes to your spiritual fitness goals, you may find great benefit in saying, "*I will* believe God for—" or "*I will* trust God to help me—" and then voice the specific goal-related choice, decision, circumstance, or situation that is facing you.

Examples:

- *I trust God* to use me in any way He wants to use me. *I will* do my best to be loving, to listen with compassion, and to offer all I can give.
- *I trust God* to help me hear precisely what He is seeking to teach me through the pastor's sermon this morning. *I will* listen as closely as I can.
- *I trust God* to reveal His wisdom to me as I study His Word. *I will* stay awake while I am reading my Bible.

Our will and faith, when activated simultaneously, are a powerful spiritual force.

SPIRITUAL FITNESS GOALS
AND TEN-WEEK CYCLES

The place to begin in setting spiritual goals is with a spiritual fitness profile. List several words that are critical to your understanding of spiritual fitness. My list includes these words: *loving/giving, obeying, forgiving, praying,* and *growing.*

Make your list *your* list. Then, identify goals related to each of the words on your list. Be very practical in your goal setting. As an example, under "Growing" I listed these behaviors that I believe are crucial for me to grow in my relationship with God and in my understanding of what He wants me to pursue and accomplish in my life:

- Have a morning devotional time every day.
- Get involved in at least one ongoing ministry activity at my church.
- Speak about Jesus to at least one person every day.
- Meditate on one verse in the Bible every day.

When it comes to my morning devotional time, I have a very clear definition for what that involves. It means spending a minimum of fifteen minutes at the beginning of every day—and ideally a lot more time than that—reading my Bible, talking to God, and listening to God. These behaviors have become habitual in my life, but at the beginning, I needed to be very intentional about these activities.

At various times, I have set very specific goals related to forgiving and obeying. I continue to have specific things about which I am praying, including a list of people for whom I pray regularly. Every ten weeks is a good time to reevaluate that prayer list and take note of answered prayers that I can convert to praises!

I also set very specific goals about how I want to give, or how I want to express love to various people during an upcoming ten-week time frame.

Since Bible reading is a critical part of my morning devotional time, I sometimes put down specific Bible-reading goals for a ten-week cycle. Or, I might identify a particular topic that I desire to study for the next ten weeks.

SPIRITUAL FITNESS AND YOUR TEAM OF 3®

It is very important that you and your Team of 3® come up with a method of accountability to one another on spiritual fitness goals. As much as possible, I encourage you to team up with two people who share your faith, and perhaps attend your church or are members of your same denomination. That way you are likely to have some mutual goals about which you can encourage one another. Some teams have set the following mutual goals:

Daily devotions:	☐ yes	☐ no
Meditate on one Bible verse:	☐ yes	☐ no
Prayer:	☐ yes	☐ no
Bible study:	☐ yes	☐ no

I talked to one Team of 3® a few years ago that had mutually agreed upon a goal of attending a noonday communion service at their church every day during Lent—the fifty days before Easter. They started a ten-week cycle on Ash Wednesday, the first day of Lent. They decided they would continue to attend noonday services for the forty days after Lent, which took them to Ascension Day. In all, they were going to be going to noonday communion services five days a week for ninety days, or twelve and a half weeks.

I thought that was a long time, and the team actually admitted to me later that the last three weeks of their commitment were the most difficult. Nevertheless, they accomplished their goal. Among the three of them, they only missed six days of attending noonday communion services. Was this spiritually meaningful to each of the team members? Very much so. They still look back on that time as being a special time of spiritual growth and development in their lives individually, and in their friendship. (This Team of 3® is still working together after four years. They just started their twenty-first ten-week cycle!)

No matter what goals you might agree upon mutually, be sensitive in your response should you note that a team member has marked *no* to spiritual fitness activity for several days in a row. Keep in mind always that your role is not to judge or condemn, but to encourage and build up. Your role is not to challenge the person's faith, but to encourage the person to pursue and fulfill their spiritual fitness goals.

I strongly encourage Team of 3® members to pray for one another—and to do so even if you are linked to people who may not share your faith or your commitment to Jesus Christ as Savior and Lord. You can always pray *for* another person, even if that person doesn't know it or desire that you do so. You should be cautious, however, in praying *with* Team of 3® members who may not want you to pray with them. Always ask before launching into a prayer.

If you are linked to Team of 3® members with whom you share faith and also have the same basic understanding of prayer, you may find that prayer is a tie that binds you very closely together. Asking for prayer from your team members may be the key to helping you through a difficult period in the pursuit of your goals, especially your spiritual fitness goals.

SPEAKING DICTUMS FOR SPIRITUAL FITNESS

As with all other dictums, you need to develop spiritual dictums that are directly related to the type of person you desire to be—the character you desire to have, the identity you want to have as a spiritual being, the relationship you desire to have with God and people who believe as you do, and the relationship you desire to have with those who don't believe as you do. Speak your spiritual life dictums to yourself daily, perhaps as part of a morning devotional time.

Possible Spiritual Fitness Dictums

1. I AM a loving person.
2. I AM serving God with my whole heart.
3. I AM a person of prayer.
4. I AM grateful for God's blessings.
5. I AM being led by the Holy Spirit.
6. I AM living the abundant life.
7. I AM meditating on God's Word.

COACH'S CLIPBOARD

I'm a coach, and coaches give their players specific exercises as a part of workout drills. So . . . here are your exercises for this chapter!

Build your core.

Exercise: Identify your core spiritual values—list at least one and no more than five. (Examples: leadership, mercy, hospitality, giving, speaking, serving, soul winning.)

Set your goals.

Exercise: Set long-term goals related to each of these values and then break them down to a set of ten-week-cycle goals.

Begin to change.

Exercise: Determine "I WILL" and "I BELIEVE" statements to go with your goals. ("I WILL" statements are related to specific behavior; "I BELIEVE" statements are statements of your faith regarding the outcome of your behavior.)

Exercise: Set "I AM" dictums for the spiritual identity you seek to develop and have. Voice them daily—perhaps several times a day.

Be accountable to others.

Exercise: Report daily to your Team of 3® about your progress toward your ten-week spiritual fitness goals.

TOTALLY FIT LIFE TRUTH

The spiritual you is the you that
steps into eternity after you die.

CHAPTER 11

Issues Unique to Men After 40

Quincy's wife came to see me. She was concerned that Quincy was suddenly acting in an erratic way—he was shopping for a red sports car and had started wearing designer sunglasses. She found a brochure on skydiving on the top of his workbench in the garage. "What's up with him?" Evie asked. "Is it a midlife thing?"

Quincy was forty-six years old, so I assured her that midlife was very likely a big part of the problem. I asked a few more questions as sensitively as I could and learned that Quincy had experienced a few "failures" in the bedroom in recent months, but he had been unwilling to talk about those failures with Evie. He had generally seemed a little depressed.

"His work seems to be going all right, but he's grumpy most of the time he's home, and I think he might be grumpy at work too," Evie said. "That isn't really like him. Quincy is usually a pretty sunny guy. I'm trying to figure out if he's sick and needs to see a doctor, or if he's just getting a little older and needs to sign up for your exercise program, or if he needs a little more inspiration and needs to get to the church more often."

I laughed. "He probably needs to do all three!"

I strongly recommend that every man have a baseline set of medical tests as he hits midlife so he will know "the numbers" he may have to deal with when it comes to working on physical and nutritional fitness. Also, a number of medical problems show up in midlife that don't reveal themselves before that time. These medical problems can sometimes be recognized in blood tests and physical exams even before the man is fully aware of more obvious symptoms.

One of the great advantages of the Totally Fit Life is that it also calls upon men to reevaluate their emotional, directional, and intellectual fitness, which gives them some help when it comes to feeling discouraged or frustrated about growing older. For many men, there's one key that fits a lot of fitness-related doors, and it's labeled "testosterone."

MAINTAINING GOOD LEVELS OF TESTOSTERONE

A slight paunch, getting out of breath after climbing just a flight of stairs, having less muscle tone, experiencing sexual problems—all can be related to low testosterone. A man who doesn't feel as fit, capable, or good-looking as he once felt is a man who can get depressed! Dissatisfaction with life—including emotional difficulties in relationships, a general malaise, a lack of ambition and direction—can spiral downward into discouragement and even depression.

Unfortunately, the relationship between depression and testosterone levels appears to be cyclical. Men who are depressed can have as much as 20 percent less than normal testosterone levels. Lower testosterone increases the probability of depression, which in turn decreases testosterone.

Medical researchers have a fairly new term for those who develop low testosterone levels: "irritable male syndrome." That may just be a nice way of saying "midlife crisis!"

The fact is that testosterone levels begin to decline slowly after a man hits age twenty, but they reach a noticeable decline in middle age.

What actually results from low testosterone?

- Muscle mass becomes harder to achieve and maintain if testosterone is low. The result is more flab.
- The brain has "testosterone receptors," and mood can be affected if testosterone is too low. The result can be more despondency.
- Low sex drive and premature ejaculation, as well as occasional impotence, can be symptoms of low testosterone. The result can be lower sexual performance or satisfaction.

Who knows how a flabby, despondent, sexually dissatisfied man will respond to life? The possibilities are mostly negative as far as I can tell.

Identifying Low Testosterone

How can you tell if you have low testosterone? Blood tests and saliva tests are available to measure testosterone levels. Saliva test kits are available through a number of sources, including online sources, for example: www.hrtexperts.com. Make sure you have a test that measures both total and free testosterone. Free testosterone—normal range of 350–1,230 nanograms per deciliter—is the most active form of testosterone. If you do a home test, you should keep in mind that testosterone levels are lower in the evening. Have a sample from both morning and evening analyzed. Numbers above 700 are preferred by most physicians.

There's also a basic questionnaire known as the Saint Louis University Androgen Deficiency in Aging Men (ADAM) questionnaire. This questionnaire asks the following ten questions:

1. Do you have a decrease in libido (sex drive)?
2. Do you have a lack of energy?

3. Do you have a decrease in strength and/or endurance?
4. Have you lost height?
5. Have you noticed a decreased "enjoyment of life"?
6. Are you sad and/or grumpy?
7. Are your erections less strong?
8. Have you noticed a deterioration in your ability to play sports?
9. Are you falling asleep after dinner?
10. Has there been a recent deterioration in your work performance?
    (Dr. John Morley: Division of Geriatric Medicine, Saint Louis
    University School of Medicine, St. Louis, Missouri 63104)

If a man answers yes to questions one or seven, or yes to at least three of the other questions, he likely has low testosterone.

In addition, men with low testosterone tend to get angry at trivial incidents and enjoy life less. Life can seem like an endless chore—an unending stream of responsibilities and obligations, rather than a joyful journey.

Ten Things to Help Increase Testosterone

The goal, therefore, for many men who hit midlife is to do everything they can to increase testosterone. Here are some of the things that have been shown to be effective:

1. *Lower the stress level in your life.* Stress can cause testosterone to drop.

2. *Stay competitive.* Even competing vicariously by cheering for a sports team can increase testosterone levels on a short-term basis. Competition does not necessarily mean a keen desire to win at all costs, which can be stressful. It also means staying ambitious, which can be interpreted "making goals and staying in hot pursuit of them." Those who take on new challenges are, in effect, competing against the lethargic or mundane status quo of their own lives. That is a health-producing form of competition!

3. *Get your weight, and especially the percentage of your weight that is fat, into the right range.* Men who are more than 30 percent above their ideal body weight tend to have a significant drop in testosterone.

4. *In losing fat, make sure that you maintain good nutrition.* Merely cutting back on calories doesn't work. Men who fast to lose weight tend to lose as much muscle as fat and they also tend to experience a period of gluttony after their so-called diet, which can be more damaging to testosterone levels than if they hadn't fasted in the first place.

The subject of fat in the diet of men past middle age is a bit tricky. A man's body makes testosterone from cholesterol. But too much cholesterol is bad for the heart. The overall recommendation appears to be that men continue to eat lean beef, lamb, low-fat dairy products, and a minimal amount of butter. Use olive oil and vinegar for salad dressings. Have a handful of nuts a day, and then stay away from stick margarines, and foods such as cookies, doughnuts, cakes, french fries, crackers, and most ready-made meals.

5. *Maintain a good balance between protein and carbohydrates.* Too much protein can actually lower testosterone levels, but so can too little, in relation to good carbohydrates found in fruits and vegetables. Try to have some of each at every small meal you have in a day.

6. *Cut out alcohol.* Alcohol, in the first place, puts the brakes on fat loss. It can also slash testosterone levels faster than the intake of any other singular substance. Over the long term, alcohol reduces the sensitivity of the testes to the luteinizing hormone, which stimulates the testes to produce testosterone. In plain language, it lowers the manufacturing of testosterone in the body.

7. *Continue to work out with weights.* Resistance or weight training is critically important for men after midlife. The great news about exercise and testosterone levels is that three or more hours of

vigorous exercise a week has been linked to increased testosterone levels—as much as an 11 percent increase! We're not talking moderate exercise here, such as walking. The exercise must be vigorous.

Some weight-training routines work better than others. Following is the most effective routine I've found in my research:

> Weight-training exercises that involve multi-joint exercises such as the leg press, bench press, seated row, and lateral pulldowns. 5 sets x 5 repetitions (with one minute of rest between sets) *Once you can do all five repetitions in all five sets, increase weight by five pounds.*

Such a routine, of course, is not one that you should start doing tomorrow. Work with a good trainer who can show you the correct technique for each exercise. Ten reps with good technique are better than forty sloppy ones. It may take you several months to work up to the maximum vigorous level required to improve testosterone levels. I also recommend that you work with a trainer who understands the importance of coupling large-muscle-group with small-muscle-group exercises.

The amount of muscle mass that is active during a resistance training session has a direct relationship to blood testosterone concentration.

8. *Don't eat too many soy products, if any.* Soy protein is sometimes recommended to middle-aged men because it has been linked to a reduced risk of heart disease and some forms of cancer. However, other studies show that it lowers testosterone levels and can disrupt normal endocrine function.

Men and women are very different when it comes to soy. Soy has been shown to have beneficial effects for menopausal (midlife) women—reducing many of the symptoms associated with menopause. Those same effects don't translate to men. If you are an avid user of protein shakes as part of your nutritional fitness program, choose a protein powder that is not soy based.

9. *Make sure you get enough zinc.* Zinc has been shown in numerous medical studies to raise testosterone levels. Zinc is found in sirloin steak, lamb chops, turkey, and oysters. If you don't eat these foods on a regular basis, then a vitamin and mineral supplement of zinc can work for you! (Take a daily supplement that has fifty or fewer milligrams of zinc. Too much zinc can interfere with the body's metabolism of copper.) A number of zinc supplements include magnesium and vitamin B6.

10. *Put your exercise emphasis on weight training, but also do some cardiovascular exercises to benefit your heart, lungs, and blood-vessel system.* Most trainers recommend about ninety minutes a week of cardio exercise (aerobics), with a day or two off between half-hour sessions. In other words, you might do thirty minutes of cardio three times a week, or forty-five minutes of cardio twice a week. You can do weight-training on the other days for a six-day exercise cycle.

Also, although exercise is one of the best ways to boost and maintain testosterone levels, don't overtrain. Keep a balance between aerobic and weight-training exercises and you'll see the result you want: an overall increase in testosterone.

Finally, don't expect to see this result after one week of exercise and eating right! Give yourself—oh, at least ten weeks.

OTHER MAJOR PROBLEMS FOR MEN

There are several other physical problems that men after midlife tend to have, but the good news is that if a person will do the ten things identified above, many of those problems will be greatly lessened or eliminated. Here are some insights, however, into several of the problems I routinely see in midlife men, but not in midlife women.

Lower-Back Pain

Lower-back problems are often linked to carrying too much weight around the waist. Eat right, exercise, and cut out alcohol, and you'll have less waist and, likely, less lower back pain!

If you have lower-back problems, check the way in which you lift items. Make sure you are stretching! Many lower-back problems are due to tight hamstrings, the biggest muscles in your body, and tight piriformis muscles, which run through the gluts. Regularly stretching these two muscle groups can greatly minimize lower back pain.

Heart Attacks and Heart Disease

Do the ten things we listed to keep testosterone levels high and you likely will be doing the very best things you can to prevent heart problems.

It is critically important that you stop smoking if you are a smoker. The link between heart problems and smoking is extremely high for both men and women, but perhaps because more studies have been conducted using men as research subjects, the link between heart problems and smoking is higher for men.

Stress is also a major factor in deadly heart attacks among those who are in midlife. Do your utmost to address stress in every area of your life. Address it physically, nutritionally, directionally, emotionally, intellectually, and spiritually!

If you have high blood pressure, work with your physician to bring it down. If you have high cholesterol, work with your physician to bring it down.

When it comes to heart health, the old phrase "less is more" often applies. Less fat, less sedentary lifestyle, less stress, less nicotine, less alcohol, less worry, less negativity, less anger, and less of just about everything you know that is bad for a person can result in more health! As always, I like to think on the positive side. Aim for *more* good-nutrition days, *more* exercise, *more* joy, *more* friends, *more* purpose, *more* relaxation and sleep, and *more* spiritual growth.

Baldness

It's only a problem if you make it a problem. I've discovered something wonderful in my years of working with the Totally Fit Life program. Most women don't care if a man is bald. Men tend to be far more preoccupied with their hair loss than women are. There's very little you can do to prevent baldness—most male-pattern baldness is predetermined genetically. Whether you choose to purchase a hairpiece or have hair implants is entirely up to you, but spending lots of money on products that are aimed at slowing or eliminating baldness is generally a waste. Keep your hair healthy and your scalp clean and you'll be fine.

Prostate Problems

Problems with an enlarged prostate gland and prostate cancer tend to show up later than midlife, but men in their forties can have prostatitis. It's good to know what's involved.

The prostate is a walnut-shaped gland in men that lies directly under the bladder and surrounds the upper portion of the urethra—a tube through which urine flows out of the body. It is about one and a half inches long and looks a little like a small doughnut with a straw (the urethra) extending from the center of the doughnut. The prostate gland produces most of the fluid that makes up semen, which is the fluid essential to reproduction.

There are three main prostate disorders: prostate cancer, an enlarged prostate (actually called benign prostatic hypertrophy or BPH), and prostatitis. A medical test called the PSA test is usually used to detect prostate cancer. An enlarged prostate has symptoms that include a weak urinary stream, problems starting and stopping urination, excessive nighttime urination, and an urgent need to urinate. Prostatitis usually occurs in men between twenty-five and forty-five years of age. Its symptoms include frequent urination, burning while urinating, painful ejaculation, excessive nighttime urination, and problems starting and stopping urination.

Studies have shown that men who eat more than one hundred grams of fat a day increase their risk of prostate cancer by as much as 50 percent! To help protect against prostate cancer, therefore, cut out fat. Avoid overeating saturated fats in meat, poultry skin, cheese, butter, whole milk, ice cream, fried foods, mayonnaise, and polyunsaturated fats found in most plant oils (including soy bean, safflower, and sunflower oil).

Those interested in improving prostate health should also take in plenty of antioxidants, such as green tea, and increase their intake of fiber. Nutritionists usually recommend the following substances for good prostate health: vitamin E, selenium, vitamin D, Coenzyme Q10 (CoQ10), and Lipic acid. Supplements helpful for those with enlarged prostates are saw palmetto, beta-sitosterol, pygeum Africanum, nettle root, and zinc.

Colon Cancer

Colon polyps and colon cancer are serious problems that tend to be associated with men in their forties. Have a baseline colon test when you hit forty and then have periodic tests after that. Colon cancer can be treated effectively, but it needs to be caught early.

Type 2 Diabetes

The best preventive steps you can take against developing type 2 diabetes are to become nutritionally and physically fit! Eating the right foods in the right intervals and at the right amounts is a formula for steady blood sugar. Exercise is also highly beneficial for keeping blood sugar levels in line.

SPEAKING DICTUMS ABOUT YOUR MASCULINITY

You *are* a man. Your masculinity is subject to your own personal definition, and in most cases, you won't need to speak dictums to yourself about your manhood. You may need to voice dictums related to specific things you seek to accomplish in response to various male-only issues. Add those dictums to the dictums you have developed in other areas of the Fitness Star.

Possible Men-Only Dictums
1. I AM humble.
2. I AM a good husband.
3. I AM filled with compassion.
4. I AM a good friend.
5. I AM forgiving.
6. I AM a good father.
7. I AM a good listener.

TOTALLY FIT LIFE TRUTH

A man is a wonderful thing to be.

CHAPTER 12

Issues Unique to Women After 40

When people come to the Totally Fit Life program, I often ask, "What brings you here? Is there a specific thing that became the triggering factor or that caused you to conclude, 'I need to be more fit' in some area of your life?"

MENOPAUSE

Carla replied to these questions very quickly and succinctly: "The big 'M.'"

"The big 'M'?" I asked. I wasn't as smart then as I am now.

"Menopause," Carla whispered loud enough to be heard thirty feet away.

"Aha!" I said.

"I know why they call it 'the change,'" she said. "It changes everything!"

"What kinds of things has it changed in your life?" I asked. "Give me some specifics."

"It's changed the texture of my skin—I have lots more wrinkles and bags and sags. It's changed my energy levels, my sleep patterns, and the way I feel about sex. It's changed the way I dress. I wear lots more loose clothing and cotton garments now because they are cooler. Hot flashes, you know. It's changed my mood—I'm a lot more prone to depression. Some days I feel as if I'm on a roller-coaster—I'm up, I'm down, I'm sideways. I'm all over the map in what I think and want and feel. It's changed some of my goals and desires. It's changed the way I plan out a day. It's changed *everything*."

"What hasn't it changed?" I asked.

"Well," Carla paused. "Let's see." More pause. "I guess . . ." More pause. "I still love God." Pause. "I still love my husband and kids—although I wonder at times if my husband still loves me, and I get irritated a lot with my kids. So they might not love me as much right now. I still like my job, at least on most days—but I have lots less patience with my lazy boss and inexperienced secretary. I still like my home and the place we live. I still like my church."

I was grateful she listed so many positives. In the years since I met Carla I've met lots of women who could hardly think of anything they truly loved or liked. Most women going through menopause take a real hit in how much they like *themselves*. When they get a quart or two low on estrogen, they also seem to get a quart or two low on self-worth.

I've discovered several things about menopause, mostly from talking to women who are facing it (premenopausal), going through it (menopausal), or have been through it a few years previously (postmenopausal).

First, women perceive and respond to menopause differently—not every woman is sad to hit menopause; not every woman is glad. The change can be welcomed, embraced, and seen as something positive, even liberating. Some women are very happy to be beyond PMS, cramps, menstrual cycles, wondering if they might be pregnant if they don't want to be, worrying that they might *not* be pregnant if they do want to be, thinking about birth control, and planning events to some degree around their periods.

Other women see menopause as a signal that they are now "old." They see it as robbing them of their youth, beauty, allure, and sex appeal. They are sorry to see their potential for childbearing come to an end. They are saddened by the changes they see in their bodies.

I've noticed that the women who feel shackled by menopause—and who don't want to go through it—tend both to have more negative symptoms and talk more about menopause as a negative experience. Those who feel that menopause is a normal part of life, and who are willing to embrace the change, tend to report fewer negative physical symptoms.

Second, I've learned every woman goes through menopause in a little different way physically. In the first place, some women hit menopause early, even in their mid to late thirties. Others don't experience menopause until their mid to late fifties. The vast majority of women experience the change in their late forties and early fifties, with as many as ten to fifteen years of premenopausal symptoms.

Some women have very few symptoms associated with menopause— a few even seem to feel better physically than they did in their twenties and thirties. Others are miserable, with frequent hot flashes, night sweats, extreme exhaustion, and emotions so fragile they continually feel like crying.

Third, most women believe that other women understand what they are going through, and that most men don't have a clue. They are probably right. I don't claim to be an expert on the subject, but I do want to share a few things that medical and fitness research say about menopause.

First, there are a number of excellent books about menopause that give women the medical facts and present various treatment options for negative symptoms. I encourage women to seek out information about natural treatments, as opposed to the normal hormone replacement therapies that many physicians seem to prescribe routinely, as if one size therapy fits all. I've seen a number of women go through menopause without taking any hormone replacement therapy—their hearts are strong, their bones are strong, and their symptoms were mild.

If someone tells you that you *must* take hormone replacement therapy in order to prevent heart problems or osteoporosis, get a second opinion. There are many things that a woman can do to improve her heart health and the strength of her bones without taking drugs. On the other hand, there are some conditions associated with taking these drugs that cannot be cured should they arise. There are often as many risks associated with taking hormone replacement medications as there are with *not* taking them. Inform yourself. Make decisions based upon a full spectrum of information and honest, straightforward discussions with your physician, a nutritionist, an exercise trainer, and your spouse.

Second, there are a lot of myths associated with menopause that simply are not true. Let me share two of the primary ones with you.

False Myth #1

You just can't lose weight or get fit after menopause. That is categorically not true. Lots of women lose weight (fat) after menopause. Lots of women get in the best shape of their lives after menopause.

False Myth #2

Taking hormones is a necessity. Again, this is *not* true for all women. Some women are candidates for hormone replacement, but even if that is the case, they do not need to take synthetic hormones. There's a category of hormones called "bio-identical" that can be prepared specifically for an individual woman's needs at compounding pharmacies. You'll need to work with a physician who understands these hormones, and go to a special pharmacy that is not located in your department store, grocery store, or normal drugstore. But these hormones do exist, and they are helpful. Furthermore, the prescriptions are ones that are tailored to your unique hormone levels and needs at any given time during the premenopausal and menopausal years, which can span a decade. The prescriptions are usually reevaluated fairly often so that you are not taking excess hormones.

In addition to bio-identical hormones, compounding pharmacies and many nutrition stores also have natural progesterone cream that can help decrease hot flashes and a natural estriol cream that can help with thinning and dryness of the vagina.

Addressing Issues Associated with Menopause

Menopause occurs when a woman stops menstruating. Some of the negative symptoms that women experience during menopause include hot flashes and vaginal dryness, which are the most common symptoms, as well as mood swings, frequent vaginal infections, cold hands and feet, night sweats, fatigue, headaches, a decreased sex drive, breast tenderness, palpitations of the heart, insomnia, drying of the skin, vaginal itching, bladder infections, dizziness, and an inability to concentrate. During a hot flash, blood vessels dilate and skin temperature rises and flushes the skin. This usually occurs about the neck and head and only lasts a few seconds to a minute.

Many of the symptoms associated with menopause are related to a lower production of estrogen in the body. Estrogen does *not* come only in medication form! Foods that are highest in plant estrogens are soy, flaxseed oil, alfalfa, fennel seeds, flaxseed, whole grains, parsley, and celery. Studies have shown that one cup of soy is equivalent to a regular dose of Premarin, a well-known hormone replacement drug. Soy flour or whole-soy products rather than soy proteins are the most efficient way for a woman to get phytoestrogens from soy. (Natural progesterones are also found in tropical wild yams.)

By the way, did you know that there's no word in Japanese for "hot flash"? Japanese women eat many soy foods, and only about 16 percent of the women in Japan and other Asian nations complain of menopausal discomfort. This is in contrast to the United States and European nations where soy foods are used less often and 75 percent of the women complain of hot flashes and other negative symptoms.

Since hormones such as estrogen and progesterone are made from cholesterol, it is important that a woman *not* go on a no-cholesterol or no-fat diet. A woman should, however, avoid hydrogenated, polyunsaturated, and saturated fats. The "good oils"—olive oil, fish oil, and flaxseed oil—should remain in the diet.

Some of the herbs helpful in controlling menopausal symptoms are black cohosh, dong quai, chasteberry, licorice root, ginkgo biloba, and genistein. Promensil is an isoflavone supplement made from red clover that may also be helpful.

On the vitamin and mineral front, studies have shown that women who are experiencing depression associated with menopause often are low in magnesium.

HORMONE-BASED MOOD SWINGS

Whether a woman is in menopause or not, a woman's body is a delicate balance of hormones at all times. A number of nutritional and fitness factors can help keep her body in balance. It is especially important that she not have excess estrogen in her system. Too much estrogen can inflame abnormal cells and have other negative health consequences. Here are some basics to check:

- Avoid exposure to xeno-hormones or xeno-estrogens, which are manmade chemicals in the environment that fool your body into believing they are natural estrogen. These chemicals are found in alcohol, fingernail polish and remover, varnishes, degreasers, dry-cleaning fluids, herbicides, emulsifiers in cosmetics and soaps, paints, industrial cleaners, glues, pesticides, plastics, and PCBs.

- Avoid xeno-estrogens in fatty beef, whole milk, butter, cheese, pork, and other fatty cuts of meat. Choose meats that are lean and dairy products that are no-fat or low-fat.
- Avoid alcohol. It can contribute to a poorly functioning liver, which impacts estrogen levels.
- Avoid excessive use of prescription medications and over-the-counter medications such as Tylenol that can place strain on the liver.
- Curb your intake of salt and caffeine.
- Make sure you eat enough fiber. Fiber helps eliminate excess estrogen through the colon. Foods high in fiber are whole grains, beans, peas, fruits, legumes, and lentils.

When you are feeling stressed, consider drinking a cup of herbal tea, such as chasteberry, skullcap, or dong quai. Also consider taking a steamy hot aromatherapy bath. Add four to ten drops of essential oils to hot water while filling your bathtub, and soak in the tub for twenty minutes. Lavender, geranium, and rosemary have especially calming effects.

OTHER PHYSICAL PROBLEMS
THAT TEND TO APPEAR IN MIDLIFE

There are several other conditions that tend to occur in women, and not as frequently in men, beginning in midlife. Let me address them in a very broad way. If any of these conditions is pertinent to your life, talk to your physician and become as informed as possible.

Osteoporosis

Osteoporosis literally means "porous bones," and about one in four women develop this condition of significant bone loss after menopause. This makes them more susceptible to bone and hip fractures, dental problems, and developing a "dowager's hump." The good news is that a number of things can be done nutritionally to help prevent or slow the development of osteoporosis.

- *Increase your calcium.* Milk and milk products are good sources of calcium. (Choose low-fat dairy products.) Vegetables such as broccoli, cauliflower, peas, beans, almonds, and sunflower seeds are also high in calcium. Just as important as your taking in calcium, you must avoid foods that rob you of calcium. Foods high in oxalic acid inhibit calcium absorption. So don't eat too much asparagus, spinach, chard, rhubarb, or beet greens. Also avoid carbonated beverages, caffeine, alcohol, and sugar. Limit your consumption of red meat.

  Make sure you have sufficient hydrochloric acid in your stomach to absorb calcium.

  If you take calcium supplements, the best ones are "chelated" forms of calcium, such as calcium citrate, calcium aspartate, or calcium fumarate.
- *Eat foods rich in vitamin D,* such as egg yolks, salmon, and fish oil.
- *Eat foods rich in magnesium* (whole grains, apples, apricots, avocados, bananas, cantaloupes, grapefruit, soy products, garlic, lemons, lima beans, and peaches).
- *Exercise!* Weight-bearing exercises and calisthenics are the two forms of exercise that stimulate the growth of new bone cells. You can buy dumbbells at a department store or athletic supply store to begin a basic weightlifting program at home.

Thyroid Problems

Beginning in midlife many women complain of feeling physically "cold" all the time—at least when they are not experiencing hot flashes! Often this is a result of a thyroid deficiency. Hypothyroidism—low thyroid levels—has also been linked to heart attacks.

The Barnes Test is a simple self-test. Immediately upon awakening in the morning, shake down a thermometer and place it under your armpit for ten minutes while lying in bed. Normal range is considered 97.8–98.2 Fahrenheit for first-in-the-morning readings. If your temperature is below 97.8, you may have a thyroid deficiency. Do this for several days since women who are still menstruating can have fluctuating temperatures. Generally the readings on the second and third days of a menstrual cycle are considered good days for the test. A woman whose temperature is consistently higher than 98.2 may be fighting an infection, even one that she doesn't know she has.

Some cancers show an increased body temperature long before more obvious symptoms appear. The thyroid gland can be stimulated naturally by taking kelp, a natural form of iodine; or if that doesn't help, there is an effective natural thyroid hormone available (as opposed to the commonly prescribed synthetic one).

Yeast Infections

Yeast, also called candida, is a single-celled organism found everywhere: water, air, and land. When yeast is allowed to "overgrow," it can affect nearly every organ in the body and particularly the GI tract, nervous system, genital/urinary tract, endocrine system, and immune system. Sometimes normal yeast bacteria in the body can put out rootlike tentacles that push through the GI tract into the abdomen. Toxic waste becomes built up in the bloodstream and a number of negative conditions can result, including fatigue, mental confusion, headaches, and depression. Sometimes the problems women think are associated with menopause are actually associated with a yeast infection. Here are the principal things a woman can do:

- Cut out sugar and all refined carbohydrates. Candida thrives on sugar, including milk sugar (lactose). Choose whole grains instead.

- Avoid foods with yeast and mold, such as all cheeses and yeast breads. Avoid mushrooms of all types since yeast is a form of fungus, and mushrooms are fungi.

- Avoid mayonnaise and mayonnaise products, as well as most condiments (including mustard, ketchup, barbecue sauce, soy sauce, pickles, sauerkraut, horseradish, and relishes). The only exception is apple cider vinegar, which contains good bacteria to fight yeast growth.

- Avoid preserved and processed meats, alcohol (especially beer), and any foods to which you have an allergy.

- Make sure you have enough fiber in your diet. Eat high-fiber foods, and if you need extra fiber, add psyllium seed, fruit pectin, oat bran, and rice bran.

- Supplements that fight Candida include garlic, goldenseal, grapefruit seed extract, caprylic acid, oil of oregano, and chlorophyll supplements (green food).

- Finally, take supplementation of lactobacillus acidophilus and bifidus bacteria to add good forms of bacteria into the intestinal tract.

Heart Disease and Cancer

Women are just as prone as men to developing heart disease and cancer. Heart attacks often don't have the same symptoms for women, however, as they do for men. There may be greater feelings of pressure and "indigestion-like" symptoms and less sharp or radiating pain. Studies are just now being done to determine all of the unique ways in which heart disease might manifest itself in women.

If you have a history of heart disease or cancer in your family, talk to your physician about the appropriate screening tests you should take after the age of forty. Take the tests recommended to you, and take them regularly. Both heart disease and cancer have much better treatment protocols and much higher "cure" rates than ever before, especially if the heart disease or cancer is diagnosed early.

In general, a woman's health after the age of forty is greatly enhanced by regular exercise, good nutrition, and a lowering of stress levels. No matter what aches and pains you may have, or that may appear as you age, stay active, keep eating right, and keep working to lower your stress and anxiety levels.

If you have goals related to ways in which you might overcome a physical ailment or negative symptoms associated with menopause, put them in the appropriate Totally Fit Life categories. I have known women who had menopause and other physical ailment goals in every category: physical, nutritional, emotional, mental, directional, and spiritual.

EMOTIONAL ISSUES THAT TEND
TO APPEAR IN MIDLIFE

In addition to physical conditions, there are two emotional issues that seem to rear their ugly heads in a special way after a woman is thirty. Sometimes these issues don't reach the acute stage until a woman is forty. I don't know why there's this delay between the time a woman has an experience and the time she is faced with the horror of it emotionally, but both research studies and my own work with midlife women tell me that the lag time is often there.

Sexual Abuse

Social science surveys have revealed repeatedly in the last several decades that as many as one in four adult women in our society have been abused sexually. That is a staggering statistic to me! Many eating disorders and other psychological disorders appear to be linked to sexual abuse early in a woman's life.

Rape and incest victims often have nightmares, severe and lingering fears, and lifelong feelings of low self-worth. Those who experience date rape often register strong emotions of shock, denial, shame, anger, and depression, as well as a degree of guilt, and these feelings can surface and resurface periodically throughout a woman's life. Every woman who experiences a sexual violation should seek all the help she can get in order to release her feelings of hurt, anger, and to come to a place of forgiveness (which, as stated previously, is not exoneration, but release).

Negative emotions associated with rape and incest can produce very real health dangers. Many autoimmune and infection-related diseases—including cancer and heart disease—can result from decades of unaddressed negative emotions. These negative emotions produce a form of physical stress that causes damage to various organs through increased cortisol levels. Ongoing negative emotions can also impact the functioning of the neurotransmitters in the brain, which results in fewer T-cells and other infection-fighting and cancer-tackling cells.

To continue to go through life without fully addressing sexual abuse is to allow enormous obstacles to remain in your path. They can keep you from achieving your Totally Fit Life goals.

Post-Abortion Stress

Many women who have had abortions live for years thinking that "nothing is wrong," and then suddenly in midlife they find themselves filled with guilt and remorse. Again, I don't know why there's a lag time between when a woman has an abortion and the day she regrets it with deep emotional trauma, but that lag is often there. If you have had an abortion and begin to experience midlife stress over that experience, you need to seek assistance from someone who can help you experience

God's forgiveness and also help you forgive yourself. Forgiveness is the only antidote I've ever seen that truly "cures" post-abortion stress.

Guilt and shame associated with any past behavior that you consider to be a sin can keep you from making and achieving Totally Fit Life goals. Address these issues in your life if they are a part of your history.

SPEAKING DICTUMS ABOUT YOUR FEMININITY

You *are* a woman. Your femininity is subject to your own personal definition, and in most cases, you won't need to speak dictums to yourself about your womanhood. You may need to voice dictums related to specific things you seek to accomplish in response to various female-only issues. Add those dictums to the dictums you have developed in other areas of the Fitness Star.

Possible Women-Only Dictums

1. I AM capable.
2. I AM forgiven.
3. I AM a good wife.
4. I AM beautiful.
5. I AM accepted.
6. I AM a good mother.
7. I AM deserving.

TOTALLY FIT LIFE TRUTH

A woman is a wonderful thing to be.

CHAPTER 13

Go Out and Win!

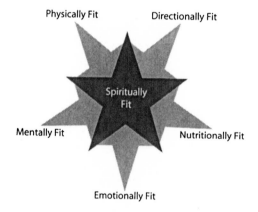

E verything up to now has been practice and prelude!" Ruth said to me. She was ready for a fresh start in her life. She was ready for the Totally Fit Life program. Are you?

I'm a coach, and coaches give pep talks before the start of any game or competition. Consider this your pep talk for the day—and for every day that lies ahead!

1. *Open up.* Stay open to the good possibilities that lie ahead for you. Stay open to the good encouragement of your Team of 3® partners and others who love you. Stay open to new information and good advice.

2. *Be supportive.* Encourage others to pursue their highest and best potential, even if they aren't in the Totally Fit Life program. Encourage your family members to join you in your quest for wholeness. Stay supportive of your Team of 3® partners. Never speak ill to them or about them.

3. *Allow for differences.* Never assume that other people are just like you in their lack of fitness or in their level of fitness. Each person comes to the quest for fitness from a different starting point and with different needs. Each person will progress at a unique rate and grow in unique ways. That principle holds true for every area of fitness on the Fitness Star.

4. *Start now.* Don't wait. Don't procrastinate. If you have a failure or you "fall off the wagon" in the pursuit of one of your goals, get up, dust yourself off, and get going again. Don't wait for Monday morning or the start of a new quarter, year, or season. Act *now*.

5. *Persist.* Stick with your goals, dictums, and good habits. Don't let the lack of interest or pursuit on the part of someone you love keep you from doing what you know is right to do.

6. *Don't obsess.* Set goals and pursue them, but don't "live" in your goals.

    In other words, don't let your preoccupation with goals dominate any given day. Don't dwell continually on today's statistics. Look for long-term trends. Weight loss, improvement in exercise routines, skill development, emotional and spiritual growth, and learning all take time and have ups and downs. Expect some fluctuations. If you focus too much on today's progress toward a specific goal, you are likely to become discouraged or unreasonably elated.

7. *Stay balanced.* Don't overemphasize any one area of fitness. In other words, don't become so preoccupied with the physical side of things (exercise and nutrition) that you neglect the emotional, mental, directional, and spiritual aspects of fitness. Don't become so introspective that you fail to address outer issues. Perhaps the greatest challenge lies in maintaining a balance among the various facets of the Totally Fit Life. You'll always need to make some adjustments. Set big goals and small ones, and keep them in balance.

8. *See yourself as a winner.* I often call people "Champion" because I am thoroughly convinced that every person has the potential to *be* a champion of his or her own life. There's great joy in winning, and part of being a champion is to see yourself as a winner and take delight in achieving the goals you set for yourself.

    Great joy comes when you do something that's difficult for you to do.

    Great joy comes when you stand up to evil or say no to temptation.

    Great joy comes when you learn something new.

    Great joy comes with loving and living in peace with others around you.

    Great joy comes when you face an obstacle and overcome it.

    Great joy comes in countless ways, on countless days, as you become more and more fit.

9. *Believe!* When you feel discouraged that you aren't making more progress and you begin to question whether you really can become fit—*yes, you can!*

    When you feel a little down that you find old habits, thoughts, and memories rearing their ugly heads once again and you wonder if you really *can* experience genuine change and growth in your life—*yes, you can!*

    When you wonder if you *can* become more fit in an area that you've struggled with all your life—*yes, you can!*

Nobody is too old, too sick, too out of shape, too fat, too *anything* to begin a fresh pursuit of the Totally Fit Life. This is the life you *want* to live. And yes, yes, a million times yes—*yes, you can live it!* Continue to believe for it.

10. *Go out and win!*

COACH'S CLIPBOARD

I'm a coach, and coaches give their players specific exercises as a part of workout drills. So . . . here are your exercises for this chapter!

Don't Wait. Start Today.
Don't Quit. Stick with the Program.
Enjoy the Journey.
Love the Rewards.

TOTALLY FIT LIFE TRUTH

Only those who give up have fully failed.

The Coach's Suggested "I AM" Dictums

Chapter 5 – Physical Fitness Dictums
First Step
- I AM physically fit.
- I AM an active person.
- I AM strong.
- I AM energetic.
- I AM healthy.
- I AM flexible.
- I AM full of vitality.

Physical Capabilities
- I AM exercising.
- I AM strong.
- I AM flexible.
- I AM agile.
- I AM coordinated.
- I AM physically fit.
- I AM powerful.

Physical Character
- I AM athletic.
- I AM an active person.
- I AM healthy.
- I AM energetic.
- I AM full of vitality.
- I AM full of life.
- I AM motivated.

Physical Self-Image
- I AM attractive.
- I AM positive.
- I AM capable.
- I AM consistent.
- I AM healed.
- I AM good.
- I AM a miracle.

Chapter 6 – Directional Fitness Dictums
First Step
- I AM achieving.
- I AM pursuing my life goals.
- I AM successful.

- I AM making a difference.
- I AM gifted.
- I AM building a legacy.
- I AM skilled.

Directional Endowment
- I AM gifted.
- I AM talented.
- I AM intelligent.
- I AM learning.
- I AM giving.
- I AM helpful.
- I AM a winner.

Directional Behavior
- I AM thoughtful.
- I AM confident.
- I AM skilled.
- I AM enthusiastic.
- I AM effective.
- I AM achieving.
- I AM successful.

Directional Application
- I AM passionate about life.
- I AM passionate about my God-given purpose.
- I AM pursuing my life goals.
- I AM making progress.
- I AM loving my neighbors as myself.
- I AM making a difference.
- I AM building a legacy.

Chapter 7 – Nutritional Fitness Dictums
First Step
- I AM eating properly.
- I AM creating a healthy body.
- I AM drinking enough water.
- I AM eating right-sized portions.
- I AM eating fresh foods.
- I AM happy.
- I AM satisfied.

Nutritional Attitude
I AM happy.
I AM patient.
I AM satisfied.
I AM positive.
I AM forgiven.
I AM energetic.
I AM whole.

Nutritional Stewardship
I AM planning my meals.
I AM making wise menu choices.
I AM buying good foods.
I AM getting proper nutrients.
I AM in control of my eating.
I AM monitoring what I eat.
I AM a good steward of my body.

Nutritional Lifestyle
I AM eating properly.
I AM eating fresh foods.
I AM eating right-sized portions.
I AM drinking enough water.
I AM cleansing my body.
I AM creating healthy cells.
I AM creating a healthy body.

Chapter 8 – Emotional Fitness Dictums
First Step
I AM joyful.
I AM faithful.
I AM a peacemaker.
I AM thankful.
I AM valuable.
I AM loving.
I AM putting others first.

Emotional Tools
I AM happy.
I AM trustful.
I AM peaceful.
I AM valuable.
I AM hospitable.
I AM kind.
I AM blessed.

Emotional Characteristics
I AM balanced.
I AM a peacemaker.

I AM a helper.
I AM a seeker.
I AM a problem-solver.
I AM a believer.
I AM a person who seeks agreement.

Emotional Lifestyle
I AM filled with joy.
I AM filled with wisdom.
I AM loving.
I AM a blessing to others.
I AM putting others first.
I AM free to love others.
I AM expressing faith.

Chapter 9 – Mental Fitness Dictums
First Step
I AM thinking pure thoughts.
I AM taking charge of my thought life.
I AM thinking about solutions.
I AM thinking monitoring my thoughts.
I AM speaking positively.
I AM learning something new.
I AM memorizing inspirational phrases.

Mental Preparation
I AM thinking right thoughts.
I AM thinking noble thoughts.
I AM thinking positively about goals.
I AM thinking about solutions.
I AM thinking about what is best for my family.
I AM thinking about what adds quality to my life.
I AM thinking about whatever is true.

Mental Lifestyle
I AM thinking about what is praiseworthy.
I AM memorizing inspirational phrases.
I AM screening my thoughts.
I AM looking on the bright side.
I AM reading uplifting books.
I AM learning something new.
I AM developing new intellectual skills.

Mental Impact
I AM in charge of my thought life.
I AM a possibility thinker.
I AM speaking positively.

I AM voicing praise.
I AM creative.
I AM a positive role model.
I AM a winner.

Chapter 10 – Spiritual Fitness Dictums

First Step

I AM a loving person.
I AM serving God with all my heart.
I AM a person of prayer.
I AM grateful for God's blessings.
I AM being led by God each day.
I AM living the abundant life.
I AM walking by faith.

Spiritual Humility

I AM forgiven.
I AM a loving person.
I AM a person of prayer.
I AM grateful for God's blessings.
I AM filled with God's Spirit.
I AM thankful for my salvation.
I AM a vessel of joy and peace.

Spiritual Student

I AM asking God for His wisdom.
I AM reading God's Word.
I AM relying upon God to guide me.
I AM listening to God.
I AM being led by God each day.
I AM thanking God.
I AM obedient to God's commands.

Spiritual Lifestyle

I AM serving God with my whole heart.
I AM walking by faith.
I AM walking in righteousness.
I AM an encourager.
I AM giving myself to others.
I AM a servant of God to every person.
I AM living the abundant life.

Chapter 11 – Men-Only Dictums

I AM humble.
I AM a good husband.
I AM filled with compassion.
I AM a good friend.

I AM forgiving.
I AM a good father.
I AM a good listener.
I AM excited about life.
I AM kind.
I AM thoughtful.
I AM a positive role model.
I AM looking for good in others.
I AM happy.
I AM in control of my feelings.
I AM responsible.
I AM calm.
I AM setting right priorities.
I AM confident.
I AM patient.
I AM passionate about life.

Chapter 12 – Women-Only Dictums

I AM capable.
I AM forgiven.
I AM a good wife.
I AM beautiful.
I AM accepted.
I AM a good mother.
I AM deserving.
I AM content.
I AM emotionally fit.
I AM whole.
I AM free.
I AM focused.
I AM a complete person.
I AM peaceful.
I AM positive.
I AM in control.
I AM kind.
I AM pure.
I AM healed.
I AM a good friend.
I AM a positive role model.

ACKNOWLEDGMENTS

To my business partner Dr. Dennis Sheehan, you are amazing. Thank you for believing in me and the vision in my heart. Long after everyone else left the field, you (a former college football center) stayed on the field with this former quarterback, until we scored. Your friendship, encouragement and support have meant so much to me. You *really* care!

To Charles Crolley who understood, felt, and then created my Team of 3® dream. Thank you for always going the second mile. You are in a class by yourself, especially every Thursday . . . and to Suzanne Crolley, your creative brilliance is remarkable.Ω

I appreciate the love and non-stop endurance of my Mom and Dad and the faithfulness of my parents-in-law, Doc and Betty. To my FIT After 50 brother, Lou and his lovely wife Robin and their children and grandchildren . . . you are all the best!

To the Pearpod design team: Jason, Doug and Kris—you guys rock.

ACKNOWLEDGMENTS

To the Cantwell family: Mike, Marie, Tim, Josh, and Benj—our two families have been joined at the hip for more than 25 years—thank you. And thanks to my entire H-A-R-V-E-S-T church family for their love; especially Jafari and Garuski.

Thanks to the entire team at Thomas Nelson Publishers, who survived this "first time" author (you have all earned push-up credits); my publisher, Jonathan Merkh, my editor, Kristen Parrish, Dr. Victor Oliver, Randy Elliot, Heather Adams, Brandi Lewis, Stephanie Newton, Greg Stielstra, Belinda Bass, and a very special thank you to JD.

To Jane Wesman Public Relations; the best PR firm this side of heaven; Jane (yes Ma'am), Lori Ames, Andrea Stein, and their entire team of PR experts.

To my close friends who have stayed in my cheering section and who have never stopped clapping through the years: Valson Abraham, Paul Engel, Bob Shank, Roger Hietbrink, Wayne Luke, Tyler and Kimi Glenn, Jerald Broussard, Dr. Brad Greene, Shelley Webb, Gil Ahrens, Jim Lane, Mark Mitchell, Michael and Kate Glenn, Phil Wilder, Dr. Frank and Mary Kay Peters, Steve Yencho, Bill McClure, Bill Dallas, Dave Dias, Chris "Shudder" Baker, Mark Garner, Tom Gordon, Dean Riskas, and finally Gerry the Barber.

To the 1990s Fitness for Life team, who were my first group of FIT After 40 success stories. Thanks for the opportunity to be your Coach. The DDG still lives on!

Finally, to my family that has endured much, so that my passion to change the way the world views fitness might be realized. To my wife Becky, aka "The Mother/Wife of All Patience," I love you so much my abs hurt...and to my children, Daniel, David and Rebekah, who can recite their dad's acronyms, quotes, and coachisms better than I can. Thanks for believing in me, but especially for trusting in the God whom we all freely serve. I love all of you beyond what I can say! Your unselfishness and sacrifices has been noted in the journal of heavenly rewards and on my "to do" list down here.

And last but not least, to my good friend and mentor, Pat MacMillian, who in 1992 suggested that I write a book . . . 1992 to 2006 . . . well, finally!

CPSIA information can be obtained at www.ICGtesting.com
Printed in the USA
LVOW081138161012

303067LV00001B/65/P